Daniel Meurois & Marie Johanne Croteau

THE GREAT BOOK OF
ESSENIAN & EGYPTIAN
THERAPIES

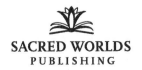

SACRED WORLDS
PUBLISHING

"Life has invented us to go to the Sun.
This is to show this path that I want to serve, nothing else."
Akhenaton [1]

We dedicate this book
To the spirit of Krmel,
To the Lake of Tiberias,
And the City of Akhetaton,
So that it has not been in vain.

With all our thanks
to Mark Medvesek, M.D.
for his caring review.

TABLE OF CONTENTS

Introduction

This book is the fruit of many years of work, research, and practice. It is also the fruit of teaching, both received and given.

It was about time for this book to come to be after many decades of contact with the invisible nature of the Universe, its energetic dimension, and its Akashic memory. This book collects the sum of acquired knowledge from a close female disciple of Christ named Salome; from Simon of the Essenian Tradition of the Krmel; and finally from Nagar Teth, who was close to Pharaoh Akhenaton.[2]

The book actually is a significant ancient database on how to approach the vibrational structure of the human body and its multiple levels of reality.

This manual contains an important corpus of therapeutic information, as well as techniques and practices for better health in order to achieve greater balance and wholeness as a person.

However, this book was not written as a simple handbook containing data and technical exercises. This study requires a mind-set reflecting the consciousness of the Sacred—the Sacred Wave of Life circulating in all of us. The therapeutic method offered here suggests a true inner approach with the knowledge of precise movements that are taught. The foundation of this approach is, of course, Compassion.

Without Compassion, each therapeutic technique described here would be reduced to a simple recipe, to a kind of mechanical procedure empty of sense and force. Then, one would be far away from the sensible and therapeutic Egyptian and Essenian priests who once structured it. And what would be the point of that?

This book is also necessary today and is deeply holistic in nature. More and more people in our Western society are rediscovering the multidimensionality of their being and, further, the Force of Life. They are the ones who learn to find their soul again—beyond a dogma—within their multiple levels of expression and connection that unifies their body. They finally rediscover again the prodigious marriage of what we call The Subtle and The Dense to create the miracle of the Living.

In this manner, the book will connect with people who are working today for a change of consciousness, becoming not only necessary but essential.

Who does this book particularly appeal to?

This book appeals not just to therapists or persons called to a healing path, but these pages will also certainly nourish anyone interested in the deep functioning of a human being, in his or her multiple levels of expression, most intimate inner-workings and in his or her relationship with the Essence of All Life. As such, it is hoped that it will be a tool used for reflection and maturation.

Those who, by discovering it, feel called by learning these therapeutic practices will obviously raise this question: "Does it require a gift to learn the original Essenian and Egyptian therapies?"

It is difficult to answer this question with a simple yes or no. What is called a gift is a natural disposition of both the soul and the body in a precise field. We can be gifted without knowing, just as we can imagine being gifted while being devoid. The answer is only given by practicing and being honest with ourselves. One thing is certain: The Egyptian and Essenian therapies will make sense, dimensional depth, and effectiveness for those who will devote themselves with heart, faith, awareness, respect, precision, and determination.

The results, therefore, will be a measure of the "alignment" of the therapist, his or her power of Love and Transparency, rather than what is called vaguely a "gift."

It is certain that for those who choose the path of these teachings, they will quickly discover that this is a path not only directed to the service of others but also an undeniable way to achieve personal growth.

We mean that it requires from the student a constant purification, a precise knowledge, humility, patience, and willingness. This is a kind of School of Life.

What will be offered to the client will undoubtedly be proportional to the work done by the therapist on him- or herself. This is not just a physical body to be healed of its symptoms. This is not just the root of its disorders to be touched and treated. His or her soul will receive a calming and evident expansion. Most of the time, it will be the beginning of a possible metamorphosis.

The ancient Essenian and Egyptian therapies impose nothing. Rather, they suggest a Light of Healing that searches for suffering at its root. They don't forbid anything and require no dogma. These therapies help those who offer them the same as those who receive them: to reveal more of themselves, to pacify and heal in depth and in full liberty.

Daniel Meurois and Marie-Johann Croteau-Meurois

NOTE:

Please understand that this book is not a substitute for a class. Practicing under the guidance of a qualified teacher will guarantee the proper assimilation of the data and the resultant expertise.

WARNING:

The authors of this book are aware that their work is already subject in whole or partially to plagiarism and numerous "borrowings" or unauthorized imitations from authors and trainers using different modalities. Therefore, they pray that readers and students in energy therapies be aware of this and use their vigilance and sense of respect.

*The data and original documents that form this book have been legally deposited with the Société Franca*ise des Gens de Lettres *before its publication.*

There is probably one hundred thousand paths that lead to the Eternal, but, one day or the other, all meet in a single point of the Heart.[1]

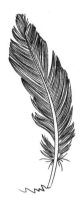

FIRST PART

At the Origin...

The origin of the therapeutic practices described in this book have undeniably been lost in the Night Ages...unless it is more accurate to say in the Sunset. For as our world approaches Sunrise, the Essenian and Egyptian therapies invite a new dawn into your life. Indeed, their luminous appearance, their simplicity, and their universality necessarily associate them with a very elaborate culture, testifying to a perception of Life "in altitude."

Our intention is not to present here the whole history, but to evoke, as a reminder, some guidelines in order to understand how they are structured in measurable time by us. Some will undoubtedly wonder about the association of the words "Egyptian" and "Essenian," which is somewhat unusual. A priori, it was not a historian who established a formal connection between the knowledge of Ancient Egypt and the Essenians. This marginal faction stems somehow from Judaism, in which the One who was to become the Christ was educated during his childhood.

To venture in this direction, we must dare to look elsewhere, where human consciousness can expand and project in an unconventional way. We mean from the side of the Akashic Annals or records, this famous Memory of Time that now holds the attention of some quantum scientists. This book was created with the help and advice of some Presences, in full mastery of their "supra-consciousness."[3]

We present to you their primary teaching, the why and how regarding the beginnings of the intriguing association between the Egyptians and Essenians.

THE EGYPTIAN SIDE

The conventional thinking about Ancient Egypt carries with it an image of a superstitious civilization that is polytheistic and, therefore, worshiping a vast number of deities or "Neters." By doing this, not only do we reduce and caricature this civilization, but we also forget too easily one of the most fascinating periods of these great people who lived by the Nile, the ones who marked the XVIII Dynasty with Amenophis III and his son Amenophis IV, more well-known as Akhenaton.

As far as we are concerned, we are precisely looking at the period when the Luxor on the eastern bank of the Nile was ordered built by Amenophis III. What the official story doesn't reveal is the primary function of this temple: a secret detachment of the ancient cult of Amon. Beyond appearances, Amenophis III indeed laid the foundations of the mystical religious reforms — above all "for initiation," which his son, Akenaton, hastened to promote as soon as he ascended to the throne. In addition, with the highly symbolic architecture expressing the energetic function of the human body, the Luxor temple contained, with its dependences, complex corridors and underground rooms. Today, these have vanished, collapsed, or been voluntarily blocked.

This architectural ensemble was intended for meetings and work for priests and therapists, who were the most initiated of their time. By order of the Pharaoh, their task was to gather and structure the essentials of the many milleniums or the wisdom of their people in the most concise and precise way in order to create a solid database to bequeath to Humanity.

Many researchers today know that this is how the Tarot was born in all of its initiatic depth. Hardly anyone, though, knows that the Tarot was the way they collected key data and procedures of their therapies.

We are obviously discussing here the therapies, which today are defined as "energy work." It was necessary to collect and synthesize these into a coherent whole, which was then dispersed and sometimes blurred. Upon the death of Amenophis III, the task remained unfinished. It was completed in the movement of the huge religious and philosophical reforms undertaken by his son Akhenaton.

So it was in the very heart of this growing city — Akhetaton — that the young Pharaoh, by adopting the Solar Ideal approached by his father, allowed the completion of an important therapeutic database. The work was entrusted to a few priests and therapists from across the Mediterranean Sea, which was under Egyptian domination at the time.[4] We know what happened to Pharaoh Akhenaton. The flowering of his reforms lasted a few years and his city was destroyed.

There exists today a fragment of the Ebers Papyrus, the most important treatise of traditional Egyptian Medicine. They mention what appears to be cancer. This treatise came slightly before Akhenaton's time. Mentioning the use of plants, it bears witness to the official part of the Tradition, its "subtle" part, which is the heart of this manual that was previously destroyed.

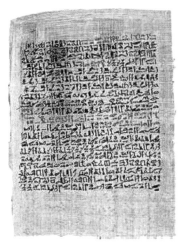

FRAGMENT OF THE PAPYRUS EBERS *(est 1550 B.C.): The most important treatise of traditional Egyptian medicine. It already mentioned what seems to be cancer. The treatise is little anterior to Akhenaton. The papyrus contains the official part of the Tradition mentioning the use of plants. Its "subtle" part, which is revealed in this book was destroyed.*

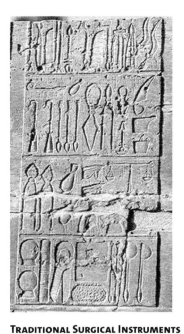

TRADITIONAL SURGICAL INSTRUMENTS TEMPLE OF KOM OMBA *The ethereal counterpart of the instruments existed in the thoughts of the initiated therapists-priests.*

The Etheric counterpart of these instruments existed in the minds of the initiated priests-therapists. The therapeutic database structured by some of these priests was no longer taught but was instead shared discretely in secret, since it constantly referred to the Unity of a Principle hardly compatible with the rehabilitated worship of Amon-Râ.

Some of the history of "subtle medicine" existing on the rolls of papyrus was then destroyed, and the teachings of the Solar Knowledge of the therapists from the city of Akhetaton became purely oral, taught by masters to disciples.

How many meanders who managed to stay alive and communicate to the priests of the young Egyptian Moses, from the court of Ramses II, is not known. The Akashic Records have not yet revealed that secret.

THE ESSENIAN SIDE

However, the Akashic Records reveal when Moses clearly received his mission, with the agreement of the Pharaoh, to take the Hebrews out of Egypt. Some of the initiated priests from the vibrational ancient therapies were part of the trip. The Records also say that Moses himself was impregnated by the unique and unifying Solar Principle that was taught to Akhenaton.

It was this manner that the therapeutic Tradition structured by Akhenaton and his father was transmitted subterraneously to the Hebrew people, or more precisely to some of their mystics. They are the ones over the centuries who would come together and define little by little a kind of distinct society, which would eventually give birth to the Essenian Fraternity. The Fraternity itself split into two groups. Some of its members chose a very ascetic, monastic existence and were known as the ones of Qumram. The other half chose a life with more freedom in small village communities. We can confirm that the famous Krmel Temple, an ancient Egyptian temple built during the reign of Amenophis III, was influenced by these two tendencies. Within the safety of the powerful walls (of the Krmel temple), the Egyptian knowledge of the initiated medicinal therapies driven by Moses and his close ones was taught to young Essenians, who were carefully selected.[5] Jeshua, still a child, stayed at the Krmel temple on a visit, which was kind of a first preparation for the role of thaumaturge that he would play later, once overshadowed by the Consciousness of the Christ. However, this is another story.[6]

A CONTINUITY

Since the resurgence of this long therapeutic Tradition, during these last decades, some people wanted to establish a difference between what appears to be, on one side, a knowledge of Essenian origin and, on the other side, a knowledge of Egyptian nature. The Tradition is not well known because the willingness of distinction generates a problem, which does not exist at the base of these therapies, and maintains a certain confusion. It is indeed a single and uniquely great Tradition, from the same corpus of knowledge that moves from one culture to another through "insiders" speaking the same fundamental language, the language of Spirit. From Essenian or Egyptian closeness, this means that these "insiders" were primarily wanderers of what has been called "The White Fraternity of Shamballa." Note that the term "white" is not related to skin color but rather to the Christ Light that synthesizes all the colors of the rainbow. That there are some slight differences in sensitivity between Egyptian priests and Essenian monks is obviously natural. More than a millennium separates them. However, both cultures shared the same understanding of Life that animates the human body regarding the relationship with the Divine, with the subtle, and also the know-how relative to the links to the Matter, the Soul and Spirit.

How did their approach slightly differ? In their more or less proximity with the physical body. To clarify, the Egyptians did not fear the contact with the body. Its touch and its life were, for them, natural, simple, and important during therapeutic treatment.

Taken in the context of the Judaic religion, the Essenians were themselves showing a more distant approach toward the physical body, sometimes hiding it under linen sheets during treatment. The only "gap" between the two ways is there and doesn't justify any kind of difference.

In addition to the procedures of the therapies, the use of oils—most anointing oils—was also shared. Both the Egyptians and Essenians attributed the same double function to the oils: to facilitate the movement of the hands on the body during some treatments and to amplify or polarize the action of the energetic Wave offered to the client. The same methods of preparation of the oils were also taught from Egypt to the land of Palestine. The principle of anointing was common.

We can affirm without hesitation that there existed a single therapeutic language used by the healer priests of Alexandria and the ones in the Krmel temple more than 2,000 years ago. The same vision inhabited them. As a matter of fact, this perception and this knowledge of the Sacred that is at the origin of all expressions of Life can only be connected to the Universal and the Timeless. We should not be surprised these techniques are coming back with force today and have a valid reason to be in our societies.

TODAY

Suffocated by hyper-materialism, a good part of our world truly aspires more and more consciously to a rediscovery of the deep laws that unify the human being to his or her subtle Divine Nature. Today is not about to go backwards; on the contrary, there is a need to expand the fields of consciousness and to go forward.

Because of the fascinating rediscovery of their therapeutic knowledge, the Essenians and the Ancient Egyptians have become naturally, some millenniums later, excellent spokespersons of this "something" within us—the existence of a sacred anatomy of the Being that seeks reconciliation. The terms of reconciliation can only be valuable to those who are sensitive to the essence and the practical content, philosophical and spiritual, of this book. All reconciliation implies the creation of bridges, communication, spaces, and exchanges.

So it must be clear that the practice in the Essenian and Egyptian therapies is not here to replace the Medicine of our time. The therapist, without exception, is not a doctor and should not attempt or give this impression. Instead, the therapist should work in concert with and under the direction of a medical professional, particularly in cases where severe pathology is present.

We must be aware that more and more doctors, even when most of the time discrete, are receptive to an approach to health including the one that is the object of this book. Working with them, therefore, will prove extremely useful, rewarding, and exciting for everyone: the doctor, the therapist, and obviously the client, whose well-being is the reason for all of this.

Life wants to give birth to worlds
but also to Itself through every one of us.

Where does the Light of an oil lamp
go when it is extinguished?

What is behind what exists?

Our project is your project.

It is the healing of the thread
that unifies all that lives, feeds, grows,
and, even, often devours.

This is the project of a therapist that makes
you artists of the health of the world.[2]

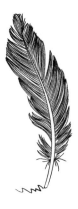

SECOND PART

The Subtle Anatomy of the Human Body

Although many concepts relating to the subtle anatomy of the human body are already the subjects of numerous books, it seems useful to review them while introducing additional information. According to the Tradition, many systems of reference exist, so much so that it is sometimes difficult to navigate when undertaking serious and coherent work in this field.

The Essenian and Egyptian therapeutic cultures are interesting because they are relatively simple to assimilate while remaining very precise. Although recognizing their existence, the Cultures do not consider the bodies beyond the causal reality of the human being. The reason is simple: The therapist is not confronted with the information directly in his or her practice.

The bodies, which the "Esseno-Egyptian" Tradition makes reference to the five bodies, which the following are:

- *The physical body*
- *The etheric or vital body*
- *The astral or emotional body*
- *The mental body*
- *The causal or karmic body*

To unify our vocabulary, here are reminders of their characteristics.

1) THE PHYSICAL BODY

Despite the complexity of its functions and the marvelous intelligence of Life expressed, the physical body is actually the less refined link that constitutes a human being. This vision does not imply, though, that it is negligible in our approach. On the contrary, it is a permanent translation and the faithful witness of a form of life and consciousness issued from the Divine.

The therapist has to address the body as a sacred construction, a true temple. This image is certainly classic to the point of being corny, but it is good to be reminded of it because all the heaviness, the imperfections, and the pain related to the physical are often the effects of forgetting or neglecting this body.

Regarding the importance that the Ancients attached to the beauty of the place, they were welcoming their clients. Beauty didn't mean wealth but rather purity. Purity implied simplicity and cleanliness both physically and mentally. The therapeutic space was indeed regularly cleaned and dedicated by an appropriate ritual.[7]

The therapist, who is aware of "what" he or she is working with, will not consider these concepts superfluous.

The welcoming of the physical person, as well as his or her comfort, is fundamental for all those who want to embrace the Essenian and Egyptian ways.

The client has to be considered a sanctuary at the very heart
of the therapeutic sanctuary.

---

2) THE ETHERIC OR VITAL BODY

The etheric or vital body is the first subtle body that defines all living beings. It is also the densest in terms of vibrations. It is so dense and closed that most of the ancient therapists viewed it as the last expression of the physical body, almost of a material nature.

For convenience, therefore, and because it is not spontaneously perceptible to everyone, it is approached apart from the physical organism, especially as it is composed of several elements of an energetic nature, even if the therapist's knowledge is not required in our therapeutic framework. Since its expression is essentially subtle, the etheric body is not endowed with a consciousness in the classic sense of the term. We would say that it acts as a relay between the higher vehicles of the being and the physical body. It is the exact warning light of the vital energy of an organism and, at the same time, its "mold." This means that from the etheric body, the density of a body is woven and takes shape. Thus, there is not the slightest cell that has not been previously formed by its etheric nature, its counterpart. Consequently, any organ of flesh owns, upstream of it, its etheric double, which transmits its characteristics and vitality.

In the course of our own journey, which results in an infinity of experimentations since most draw back Time, it is understood that the etheric body preexists before the physical body. It is the closest matrix. This is why the therapist first connects to the etheric organism of a client—in order to be able to interact positively with his or her state of health.

The connection and knowledge of the etheric are the first base of the work recommended here. It will be in vain to treat the subtler realities of the human body if, in a therapeutic context, the connection with the etheric is not efficient...except to be a born miracle performer (thaumaturge)!

Continuing to deepen our study of this body is necessary because knowing the etheric is the exact double of the physical, "on another wavelength," is not enough. It is essential to understand that the etheric body, a body by itself, is crossed by a network of highly complex energetic channels, which somehow constitute both the blood circuits and the nervous network. These channels are traditionally called the "Nadis."

To a certain level, they can be related to the meridians in Chinese acupuncture. The function of the Nadis is to distribute the subtle, vital energy—including the Prana—throughout the body. Their crossings in some precise areas of the body create points of force. (As we will see, this knowledge is required to implement the practice of the Essenian and Egyptian therapies.)

The network of the Nadis finally connect these centers of force – or major plexixes – that are the chakras, distributed through the dorsal axis. A good understanding of the nature and role of the Chakras and the Nadis is essential in the application of the studied therapies that we will return to later in much greater detail.*

Finally, note that the etheric body is the only one of our subtle bodies that is outside of our physical body. It envelops the physical exactly like a glove whose thickness is an average of two to three centimeters (around 1"). Beyond this zone, the etheric aura is its luminous extension. This aura is also noticeable by a few centimeters' thickness. It manifests in a radiance of blue gray, slightly silver sometimes.

It is important to be aware that it is not the etheric aura that the therapist is going to work but rather the etheric body. The aura is only the radiance of the body, a significant radiance because it is one of the indicators analyzed during a full lecture on the energetic organism.

* See p. 25 and following.

3) The Astral or Emotional Body

Contrary to the etheric body, the astral body is inside the physical body. It takes exactly the form of the physical body as well.

We can say it is the first of our subtle bodies to be part of this vibrational reality of "multi-layers" called the "Soul." The astral body is the center of our emotions, of our sensitive world of ourselves in the affirmation of our personality.

Therefore, we can agree that it is the theater—life after life for the vast majority of us—of a great number of events and "energetic tempests."

It is permanently under construction, since it serves as a place of refinement for our sensibilities and talents.

The therapist will have to know that, like the etheric and physical bodies, the astral body also has separate organs that are palpable on their own levels. Each of these organs plays the role of a "pre-matrix" in relation to the etheric organ to which it corresponds. The same goes for the Nadis and the Chakras.

It is always the subtle that weaves the fabric of the dense...

When we understand it thoroughly, we realize better why a suffering emotional state can affect the functioning of an organ or an astral system, which transmits the information to its etheric counterpart, which then communicates to its physical extension.

The Egyptians and the Essenians, who had perfectly grasped the principle of how this information moved similar to a bounce, structured their therapies accordingly. Mainly, they always looked to raise the level of their treatments as close as possible to the source of the malfunction.

There are types of emotional states stemming from character traits and behavioral attitudes that obviously affect in a special way some systems regulated by the Chakras. The links have been analyzed and are presented in a summary table with the Archetypes in this book.*

Regarding the emotional aura, the one of the astral body, it is naturally projected from the inside toward the outside of the physical body on a periphery, sometimes up to one-and-a-half meters (4'11") but more generally limited to a meter (3'3"). This is the most spectacular aura, comparable among some people to the veritable palette of a painter. The slightest fluctuations in mood, state of mind, or characteristics of the temperament of the being are expressed spontaneously in it. We can read in this aura predispositions, qualities, and weaknesses.

4) The Mental Body

As the name indicates, the mental body is the center of brain activity of the incarnated being. It is also inside the astral body. In this more refined combination, the

* See The Archetypes on p. 172 and p. 173. Also see p. 170.

human being becomes able to express his or her "I, Me and Myself," to individualize him- or herself, and to develop consciousness, thus separating progressively from the soul-group forcing gregarious behaviors upon the individual. Contrary to the two previous subtle bodies, the mental body does not closely fit the form of the physical body, whose purpose is to animate.

Its outlines are less defined, more vaporous, more subject to deformations that occur at the pace of the characteristics of the "cerebrality" of the person. The proper functioning of the mental body has a direct influence on intellectual capacities, some aspects of learning, and the ability to memorize. This affects each of us.

At the level of the mental body, we do not strictly speak about the existence of organs or a network of Nadis or Chakras. When discussing it, there is instead a question of "zones of sensitivities" that may affect important parts of the emotional, etheric, and physical bodies. These zones of sensitivities have the specific task of generating "energetic waves" by causing discharges in continuity or in the rhythm of brain activity more or less significant to the being.

When these repetitive discharges occur for a long time, they finally generate "Thoughts-Forms." These are energetic clusters inhabited by a specific thought, presence, or event. A thought-form can be constructive, but the therapist will focus on detecting and deactivating those that are clearly toxic.

The toxicity of some Thoughts-Forms is so great that the energetic mass can indeed weaken, like an infection, the mental then the astral body and finally the etheric body at a precise point, organ, or system. When the etheric body is reached, a function disorder or disease appears. In many cases, a harmful thought-form represents a real focus of infection where different layers of the subtle organism become unsynchronized by seeding a dysfunction or serious disorder.

Below are two examples showing how Thoughts-Forms can be perceived in the mental space of the aura.

It is extremely important to understand that the human body is able "to think in his or her head" and also "think in his or her heart" and "think in his or her belly." Some cultures and languages specify these three areas in their vocabulary and idioms. Recent scientific research has even proved that the intestinal wall contains hundreds of millions of neurons!

During the course of brain activity, there will be such-and-such zones of sensibilities of the mental body that will send their "trains of waves"—often from the Thoughts-Forms—directed to the emotional and then the etheric body. Regarding the mental aura, it is, of course, the direct expression of the activity of the mental body. It can manifest around the outside of the emotional aura at a distance of about one meter eighty (6'5") or even two meters (6") beyond the physical. It is also easily perceptible in the form of a global yellow mist. The nuances of this yellow change from acidulous to yellowish mixed with gray. Besides the Thoughts-Forms, a sensitive therapist will instantly perceive small, luminous lines. They are the mark of the "trains of waves," which we just discussed.

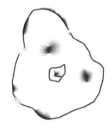

CLASSIC TYPE OF THOUGHT-FORM: *Similar to a cell with its nucleus, cytoplasm, and membrane. The membrane is more or less thick and porous, depending on the nature and age of the thought-form.*

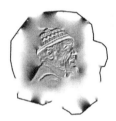

EXAMPLE OF A THOUGHT-FORM OF LONG DURATION: *The nucleus reflects a presence that, like a fixed idea, pollutes the mental space. The obvious porosity of this energetic mass shows its activity.*

In light of all this, it is easy to see that the health of a being is the result of his or her multidimensional reality. It is about chain reactions, the transmitting of information either by structuring or destructing from one body to another.

---

5) THE CAUSAL BODY

Descend now even more within the human being. Inside the vibrational reality of his or her mental body exists another: the causal body. In its manifestation in an incarnated individual, the form of energy of this body is nothing like the appearance of the human form. It is more like an envelope of ovoid light, and the spark is located precisely in the heart.

As its name clearly indicates, its body is one of the causes—namely, the seat of deep memories. Its energetic dimension triggers all mechanisms of the karmic baggage of every human being. Thus, it contains the information source that is at the origin of what we are and why we are submitted to such-and-such circumstance and hardship. The causal memory, then, affects all the layers of being. It is like a subtle game of cards we have to play during our lifetime.

It goes without saying that the recognition of the existence of the body presupposes that the therapist of the Essenian and Egyptian therapies accepts the reality of the Law of Reincarnation, or at least considers it a serious possibility. The most advanced therapies of the present method are indeed based on the action of the causal dimension within the global health of the human being. They will sometimes aim to detect the nature of a disorder of karmic origin when it manifests in

*See p. 40.

order to provide forces and tools to the client to either defuse it or better cope with it. The seed cell of this body is located, as mentioned earlier, precisely in the heart, all of the dimensions reunited. The Tradition naturally gives it the name "seed-atom." Anatomically, it is connected to the left ventricle of the heart. This atom is made of pure Akasha.* It must be seen as the absolute memory of all forms of life in terms of thinking and consciousness of itself.

In other words, it is the central bank of a being's database since the blossoming of his or her individuality. It is also the stem cell that relates directly to his or her Divine origin.[8]

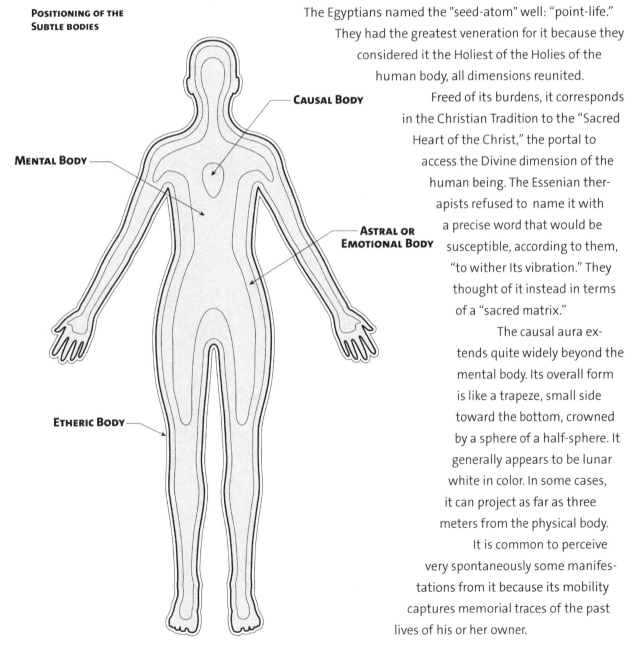

POSITIONING OF THE SUBTLE BODIES

CAUSAL BODY

MENTAL BODY

ASTRAL OR EMOTIONAL BODY

ETHERIC BODY

The Egyptians named the "seed-atom" well: "point-life." They had the greatest veneration for it because they considered it the Holiest of the Holies of the human body, all dimensions reunited.

Freed of its burdens, it corresponds in the Christian Tradition to the "Sacred Heart of the Christ," the portal to access the Divine dimension of the human being. The Essenian therapists refused to name it with a precise word that would be susceptible, according to them, "to wither Its vibration." They thought of it instead in terms of a "sacred matrix."

The causal aura extends quite widely beyond the mental body. Its overall form is like a trapeze, small side toward the bottom, crowned by a sphere of a half-sphere. It generally appears to be lunar white in color. In some cases, it can project as far as three meters from the physical body. It is common to perceive very spontaneously some manifestations from it because its mobility captures memorial traces of the past lives of his or her owner.

The image of the Perfect dwells in us for all eternity, and our only wrong is to have forgotten it. Invite this truth: The Divine, alone, is totally at home within each of us.[4]

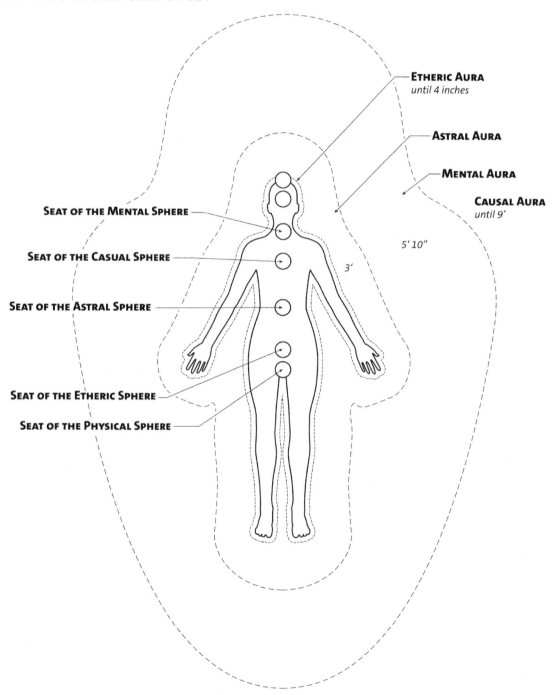

ETHERIC AURA
until 4 inches

ASTRAL AURA

MENTAL AURA

CAUSAL AURA
until 9'

5' 10"

3'

SEAT OF THE MENTAL SPHERE

SEAT OF THE CASUAL SPHERE

SEAT OF THE ASTRAL SPHERE

SEAT OF THE ETHERIC SPHERE

SEAT OF THE PHYSICAL SPHERE

DIFFERENT AURAS AND SPHERES OF ACTIVITY OF THE CHAKRAS

6) THE CHAKRAS

As the Oriental mystics, the Ancient Egyptians and Essenian insiders were fully aware of the existence of the Chakras, these major centers of energy, or plexuses, which are divided throughout the spinal cord. They were given the names "wheels of fire," "lamps," or even "altars." In the same way as their Hindu and Himalayan homologues, they enumerated them seven. However, the Akashic Records indicate that the Christ revealed to his closest disciples the existence of an eighth Chakra, Tekla, which is manifested outside the body, about fifty centimeters above the skull.[9]

For therapists, a good knowledge of the system of the Chakras is required. In fact, each Chakra represents not only a center of energy, extremely powerful, connecting to all the bodies of the human being, but it is also a vibratory reality reflecting all the energies circulating in the cosmos. Thus, each Chakra is constantly supplied in the Prana and Akasha: two essential elements for the maintenance of Life and Its Intelligence.*

According to the Essenians and Egyptians, each Chakra plays a receptive role on the back of the body (it looks like a funnel penetrating) and an emissive role on the front, where it evokes a fountain.

Whether emissive or receptive — namely, letting the energy of Life penetrate the organism or push it toward the front — any Chakra manifests in its center a sort of "pistil" more or less radiant and dynamic that enables us to easily detect its presence in the back as well as the front.

HORIZONTAL CIRCULATION OF LIFE ENERGY BY A CHAKRA (FUNNEL AND PISTIL)

The presence of the pistil, which is in fact the mark of a channel, contributes to what a Chakra would inevitably be compared to a flower. All the Traditions we are referring to here have seen that each of these flowers has a different number of petals (likewise as it is from one Chakra to another), and each petal has its own function within the vital, emotional, mental, and even causal plan.

Continuing with the image of flowers, which open more or less to receive light and then offer their beauty and perfume, the Chakras are more or less blooming into a being. They are the major witnesses as to the state of health of a person, on both the physical and psychological or spiritual planes.

* See p. 37 and p. 40.

Learning to identify the level of functioning of a Chakra by aura reading or, more easily, by "Etheric Palpation" is, therefore, one the basic tasks* of the therapeutic method discussed in these pages.

To the most sensitive of us, a Chakra is observed flatly in front during an aura reading, and it looks like a diaphragm of a camera with an iris. Each mobile element of this diaphragm is comparable to the petal of a flower.

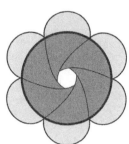

THE SHAPE OF A CHAKRA IS THAT OF AN IRIS DIAPHRAGM.

As it opens, its external petals inflate. Here is a Chakra well deployed.

The Tradition commonly accepted today allocates a color to a Chakra. Essenian and Egyptian knowledge agree with this perception. However, they would go beyond it, teaching, in fact, that each Chakra can be seen with any of the seven colors of the rainbow, depending on the level on which it is "read."

According to them, each plexus expresses and occupies a function at the level of each of the bodies of the average incarnation of a human body.

It is important to understand that the table listing the colors of the Chakras describes what is perceived classically on the etheric level. We could establish a similar table illustrating the radiance of the Chakras from the astral level, mental plan, etc.

The ancient therapists from Luxor, Akhetaton, Alexandria, and the Krmel claimed that we can psychically penetrate into the heart of a Chakra and so discover, according to the investigated level, the succession of revealed colors corresponding to the one associated with the Chakras, from bottom to top, in their etheric expression. To give a concrete example, this means that if the base Chakra is defined with the color red according to the classic Tradition, we can perceive it, when leaving the etheric level, in orange, yellow, green, and so on. If the therapist doesn't see clearly the use of this information in practice, his or her knowledge will enable a greater and more accurate understanding of the whole of the Universe that represents a Chakra. The Sense of the Sacred and Its approach toward the multidimensionality of the being will be fortified.

To finish with a quick overview of the Chakras, it is important to know that each one of them is linked to a precise endocrine gland. From there, we can understand that the dysfunction (proven or suspected) of one of the glands in the organism of a client will automatically invite the therapist to focus on the related Chakra. The reciprocal is also true. It is imperative to consider the fact that a Chakra is the director element of any system regulated by the functioning of an endocrine gland. It is the essential link between the highest vibrational levels of the being, the physical body, and the Principle of Life.

* See p. 53.

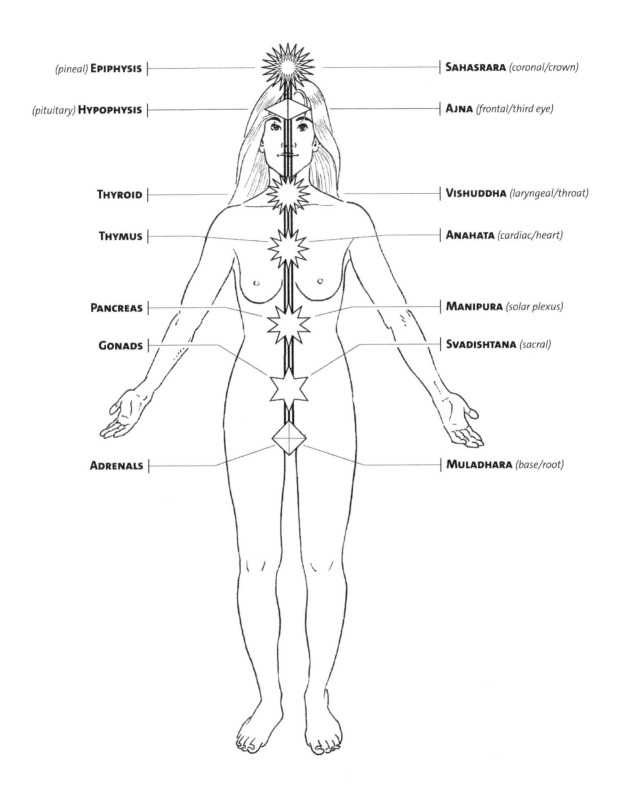

(pineal) **EPIPHYSIS**

(pituitary) **HYPOPHYSIS**

THYROID

THYMUS

PANCREAS

GONADS

ADRENALS

SAHASRARA (coronal/crown)

AJNA (frontal/third eye)

VISHUDDHA (laryngeal/throat)

ANAHATA (cardiac/heart)

MANIPURA (solar plexus)

SVADISHTANA (sacral)

MULADHARA (base/root)

CORRESPONDENCE TABLE OF THE CHAKRAS AND ENDOCRINE GLANDS

7) THE NADIS

Generalities

We turn now to the study of the Nadis. As a reminder, the Nadis are the channels through which the Energy of Life flows in the subtle bodies. The Essenians and Egyptians enumerated about 125,000 Nadis. This figure varies, though, from one tradition to another.

It is obvious that these channels, the Nadis, are a bit comparable to blood vessels, though they are not all of equal importance. Their "grade" is variable depending on their location and the role they play. So on the energetic plane, they are similar to true arteries, others to veins, and still others to simple vessels or even capillaries. They are a huge supply network spread out in a complex way that is very precise and logical within the totality of the subtle organism. The therapist will approach them at the etheric plane.

At the origin of the Nadis, we find the Chakras. They are like the "nervous extension" with multiple ramifications. In fact, it is the Chakras-Nadis connection that enables the structure of an etheric body to become a coherent "mold" from which the physical organism emerges and then develops. We can easily understand from this that the condition of the major Nadis of a being or a percentage of them will impact the state of a person's health. Accidents, surgeries performed poorly, bad breath, an unbalanced diet, and, in general, an unhealthy lifestyle often affect the Nadis. Additionally, like a blood vessel or even a nerve, a Nadi can indeed be cut and become porous and dirty, sometimes causing many various consequences.

The widest possible knowledge of the network of Nadis is consequently essential. The therapist must memorize the major ones. We just mentioned the concepts of breaking, porosity, and contamination. However, it should be noted that we have done this out of convenience. In reality, if we want to analyze the Nadis in depth, we must understand that they are not strictly "ducts" through which vital energy flows. The Nadis are the mark left by the Current of Life, which travels a multitude of ways into the etheric organism. They are, thus, the Prana in direct action and not a "fluid" circulating in a sort of sheath.

It is a more or less good "quality" of this form of Light that ensures its flow can generate a kind of "crust" on its surface.

When the crust is polarized toward the inside of the pranic flow, it results in an effect of dirt accumulation within the etheric organism. So, over time, this crust continues to grow to the point of polarizing toward the outside of the pranic flow. It is losing its used "matter" and creating waste. This waste is called an etheric slag. These slags are expulsed by the subtle organism and leave grayish imprints in the etheric aura.

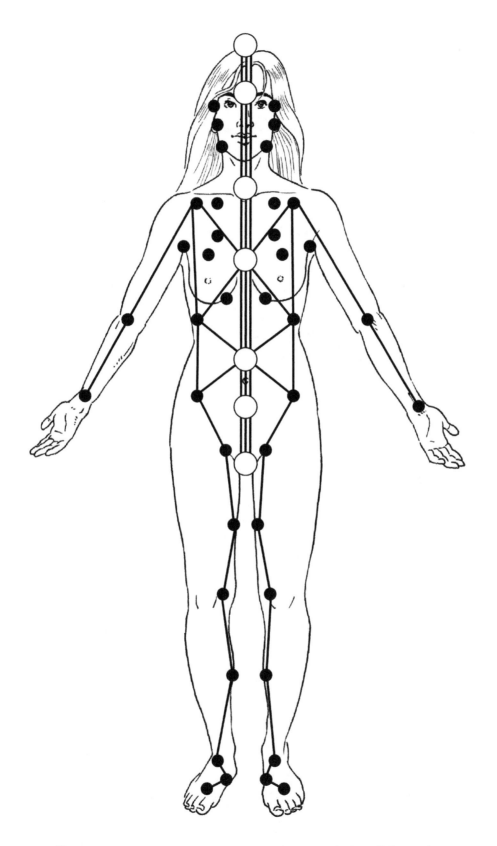

MAP OF THE MAIN NADIS OF THE HUMAN BODY, MAJOR AND SECONDARY CHAKRAS.

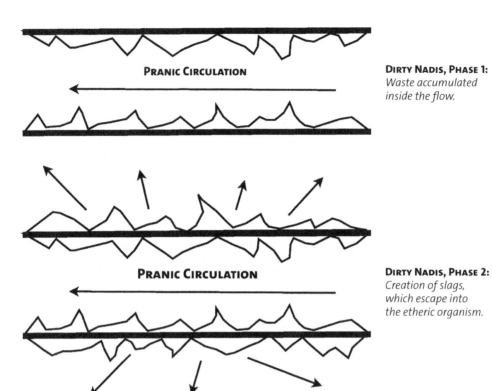

PRANIC CIRCULATION

DIRTY NADIS, PHASE 1: *Waste accumulated inside the flow.*

PRANIC CIRCULATION

DIRTY NADIS, PHASE 2: *Creation of slags, which escape into the etheric organism.*

We must also know that stress and anxiety act upon the quality of the Prana in circulation in an organism, and as such, they participate in the creation and proliferation of etheric slags. This is why cleansing and a good centering of the vital body is often beneficial before undertaking a therapy. Several methods of action will be indicated on the following pages. It is important to put them into practice before starting some treatments in-depth.

Ida, Pingala, and Sushumna

Let us focus now on three major Nadis, well apart from the others. These are the most important indeed. We are talking here about the ones that are on the dorsal axis. Regardless of the names given by the ancient therapists around the Mediterranean, it is easier for us to choose the ones that the Orient passes on to us, the ones we have already adapted over a few decades: the Ida, Pingala, and Sushumna. They form a trinity. Ida is a lunar polarity, or negative. Pingala is solar, or positive. And Sushumna synthetizes both and transcends them. Note here in passing that the terms "negative" and "positive" in this context impart no value of judgment, no more than the negative or positive poles of a battery. In this understanding, we are referring to how the Energy of Life in all its aspects is assimilated by the human organism.

You will notice that this cosmic or Divine Energy—which unifies the solar and the lunar—penetrates at the top of the skull and goes down into the body by the Sushumna. The intensity of the penetration depends on the more or less conscious awakening of the being, as well as his or her karmic baggage. The descent of this major Current of Energy or Light is fairly fluid based on the state of dilatation of the Sushumna and the encountered Chakras.

Arriving at the base of the spine, the Divine Current nurtures or stimulates the first Chakra of the being and its famous reservoir of Force called Kundalini. At this point, the Current splits in two parts. In other words, it repolarizes to go up the dorsal axis simultaneously in its left channel, Ida, and its right channel, Pingala. In their ascension, the lunar force, Ida, and the solar force, Pingala, are inevitably going to meet each time at the Chakras, from which they will receive their stimuli. Upon reaching the top of the skull, the flows of the ascending energies Ida and Pingala then spurt up and create a kind of luminous fountain easily perceptible in an aura reading. The power and "caliber" of this fountain will express the way the Force of Life is able to go through the whole being.

As indicated in the diagram, we need to be aware that the Chakras are touched and "worked" by the two vertical streams circulating permanently in the three major Nadis of the subtle organism.

And they are crossed, also continuously, from behind to the front and horizontally by a Force of terrestrial nature. This Force, equally Divine and globally pranic, is not simply telluric in the broadest sense. It is charged as well with a multitude of "trains of waves" resulting from all sources of energetic pollution created by human activity, as well as "vibrational materials" related to meetings and events in life.

We can see here how the Chakras and Nadis interact according to the circulation of the complementary lunar-solar vertical and horizontal Currents. A being's

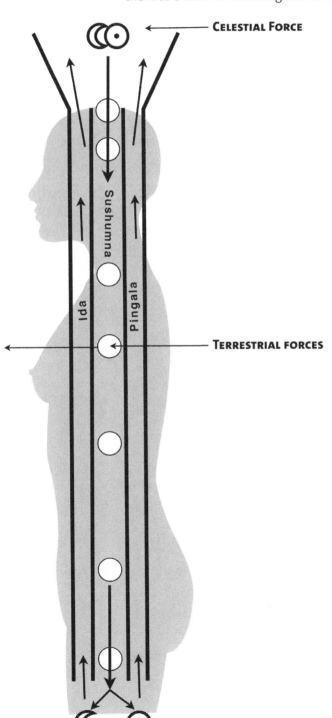

CELESTIAL FORCE

Sushumna

Ida

Pingala

TERRESTRIAL FORCES

health is relatively established by how the person "manages" the pursuit of growth both vertically and horizontally. This is where free will and the willingness of each being intervenes, including causal necessities.

Depending on the evolution of the consciousness of each person, it is obvious that the central axis, Sushumna, is called to expand. Simultaneously, Ida and Pingala will begin to "undulate" increasingly until intersecting, where they will then generate a circuit of ideal functioning, which represents the classic presentation of the subtle anatomy, schematically evoked by the Caducean symbol of doctors. Contrary to the belief of some people regarding the awakening work by the Energy of Life along the triple dorsal axis, the Chakras do not deploy one after the other in the order they are distributed in the body (namely, from bottom to top). Thus, for instance, a human being can manifest a cardiac Chakra very openly and harmoniously and, at the same time, present a deficient second Chakra. The deploying and balancing of the Chakras have nothing to do with the type of logic that could a priori be ours. They operate according to our inner growth—in other words, our intimate comprehension of Life, our relationships with others, our behaviors facing events, and the power of the Heart, in the spiritual sense.

When disorders and disease are installed in the body, we must see them like red signals flashing on a dashboard. They invite us to look for, on one hand, what level of our being they are alerting us to and, on the other hand, what the nature is of the energies we are offering to our being on the respiratory, dietary, emotional, mental, and spiritual planes. In general, the Egyptian and Essenian therapists estimated that the vast majority of health disorders start from a weakening of the soul across all layers, a poisoning reverberating through multiple desynchronizations that engender each other. They were talking of a deficiency of Love in the being.

---

8) The Secondary Chakras or Sub-Chakras

To conclude our discussion of the subtle anatomy of the human body, we must address the subject of the energetic points that the Ancients named the Secondary Chakras or Sub-Chakras.

We recognize that the designation may be questionable to the extent that the points have neither the function nor the power of the Chakras as such. We have chosen to keep it because these areas in question present themselves in the form of small vortices more or less bright in the etheric aura. They attest to their importance.

Referring to the simplified map of the subtle lanes going across the human body,* we immediately notice that what we call Sub-Chakras are points resulting from the confluence of large Nadis. On the subtle plane, they act like "doors" or * See p. 29.

"valves" more or less opened by regulating the flow of the Energy of Life in the body. Is it necessary that these "doors" be fully opened in a healthy person? Yes. Conversely, it is easy to understand that any injury, disharmony, or disease generates "energetic retentions" and contributes to some Sub-Chakras contracting gradually to the point of becoming obstructed. This is why most of the therapeutic protocols described in this manual often address these points. Knowing the map of the large Nadis of the human body well will lead automatically to an easy approach to these Secondary Chakras.

As we shall see, it is mostly physical actions that will be performed on them using simple pressure or massage with a finger precisely and locally. The massages can be performed two ways:

- Clockwise, to energize and bring the Prana in an area.
- Counterclockwise, to "open a door" by dispersing accumulated energetic waste.

The Essenians and Egyptians obviously didn't use the term "clockwise" or "counterclockwise."

They talked of "swirling" or "de-swirling" in reference to the movement of the fast evacuation of water by a circular opening in the Northern Hemisphere.

Some might be surprised by intervening on the subtle organism by pressuring the physical body. However, we need to remember—as we have mentioned previously—that the etheric is extremely close to the physical. It literally penetrates it by means of the blood. The blood is then the tangible vehicle of the subtle and sacred Energy circulating in a being.[10] Requesting a blood flow at a given point is inevitably calling for a "reinforcement of the Prana" at the etheric level.

Important Note: *The intellectual knowledge of the location of the principal Sub-Chakras is an essential requirement but will not be enough for the therapist. He or she should sense tactilely to find each of them in the body, like the way acupuncturists proceed.*

At the level of the Sub-Chakra, the skin indeed presents a slight depression and creates a "different" sensation under the pressure of the finger of the therapist. This pressure can be a little bit painful for the client. A way to find the location of the point is to perceive a strengthening of the skin and generate a small pain in the area, which supposedly nests the presence of a Sub-Chakra. It goes without saying that any pressure from the finger should take into consideration the sensitivity of the client and be measured in order to avoid any tension and resulting discomfort.

The Essenians and Egyptians were known for the gentleness and harmony of their therapeutic practices. Let's be faithful to their spirit.

**What it pulses to the deepest of our chest
is a stranger to normality. The miracle
of what it is living in you, of what loves
and of what hopes, even the shadow
of the silences, it is all but normality.**[5]

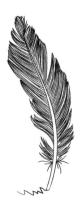

THIRD PART
What Is the Energy of Healing?

1) ITS GLOBAL NATURE

All those who are interested in energy therapies or who practice them are necessarily faced with this question: What is the identity of the force we call on to invest in our hearts and then go through our hands to help others? Where does it come from precisely, and what is it made of? To simplify the response, some are going to say it is a universal energy. This is a way to extract the principle of healing from any system of belief potentially dogmatic, which is not a bad decision in itself, since it brings back all to the intimate functioning of nature.

Others, though, will choose instead to speak of Divine energy, opting then for belief in a higher intention by an approach much more mystical. For them, this is the connection with the Divine. It is cultivated by inviting purity in ourselves. The Egyptians and Essenians obviously belonged to this category of therapists-mystics, since their practices were clearly in reference to the existence of a luminous, principled universe, a provider of absolute love, and therefore total harmony. However, they probably would not have rejected as much the idea of a universal energy reflecting the working secrets of nature.

Indeed, for those of them who were the most introduced into the mysteries of their art, within the cosmic sense, the Divine and nature were one. They viewed nature as tangible—capable of capture by our five senses—like the body of the

Divine, a body whose function was to welcome us to a matrix in which we needed to grow. They conceived of this natural body as the expression of the more dense, the more raw of the Divine reality. Behind tangible nature, they saw two others, the soul of the Divine and then the one of its spirit. In their eyes, any form of life evolved consequently within a sort of sacred ocean of Trinitarian essence.

From there, it is not about belief or not. We can't escape from the "Divine context" because we are immersed in It, and the Divine is one with nature and its most mysterious laws.

As we are living within the Divine, this means that the Divine is offering itself continuously and inviting us to rise and become closer to It, to decode It, to read It at Its levels of manifestation, visible and invisible.

The ancients created a system of thought and an approach to the therapeutic arts based on a Trinitarian understanding of the energy of healing—or, more simply, the energy of life.

According to this system, which is introduced in these pages, this energy of healing is the result of the union, in variable proportions, of the three following elements or principles:

- **The Ether**
- **The Prana**
- **The Akasha**

2) THE ETHER

Let us start by looking at the Ether, since it constitutes the mold and the energetic engine, the most basic of all we can perceive. It offers vital energy in the most concrete sense of existing. The Ancient Ones said that the Ether is composed of four distinct levels or states, each with a specific function. It is always interesting to learn about each of them.

a) The Chemical Ether: It allows the assimilation of food. It is therefore present at the level of secreted juices in the body during the process of digestion. This Ether is the densest. The Ancients said this Ether is closely connected with the Leading Intelligences of the **Earth Element**.

b) The Reproductive Ether: Its function is to cause the pulse of life, based on the "fuel" that represents the precedent. By definition, it is the one that provides the body with its physical strength and reproductive potential. We associate it with the Intelligences of the **Water Element**. It is particularly active at the levels of the blood and urinary system—especially the kidneys—as well as everything that relates to the functioning of the genital system.

c) The Luminous Ether: It rules all of our sensory functions. The breath of sensitivity is generated from it. This breath is manifested in the form of heat. The detachment of its energetic layer is perceived very clearly at the precise moment of death. This is why there is often the very clear perception of an indeterminable "light" abandoning the body at this moment. This Ether's function is to maintain the Flame of Life from the born motor of the combination of the two first Ethers. The Ancient Ones associated it with the Intelligences of the **Fire Element**.

d) The Mirror Ether: This Ether is so named because of its ability to store information generated by the physical world. Its function is to memorize everything that is derived from density and to maintain a certain cohesion of the form. It is the support for what we call today cellular memories. We traditionally associate this Ether with the **Air Element**.

These four expressions of the Ether represent what the Egyptians and Essenians called the Body of the Divine in His subtle aspect. All sensitive beings perceive an overall bluish color, slightly iridescent. From there, ancient therapists maintained that the blue color expresses the incarnation process and translates the basic presence of an organized life.

We must now understand that the Ether is present everywhere in our tangible world. It permeates all. We breathe, we eat, we feel, and we bathe in it every moment.

The Ether is thus analogous to amniotic fluid, a liquid that admits within it, in various proportions, one of the other components of the life force. The other component is the Prana.

---

3) THE PRANA

A little like the Ether, the principle called Prana is expressed in four vibratory layers. It is generally believed that the Prana is assimilated, especially by breathing. The body absorbs it in multiple ways: by food, of course, as well as through body hygiene and a balanced physical workout, but also by the nature of our emotions, by our affective world, by our thoughts, and finally, by our spiritual concerns. There are indeed four ways to receive and polarize the Prana in the body—namely, four ways to "color" it, then to assimilate it more or less well.

Before going further, it seems important to emphasize the fact that the Great Tradition, to which we refer, spoke of the Prana as the *Energy of the Soul of the Divine*, parallel to the Ether, which, let us recall, was seen as an expression of the *Body of the Divine*. Talking about the Soul leads to the personality and, by extension, to the ego in a human being. When this principle is accepted, it is easy to understand that these are the distinguishing characteristics of an ego—in other words, a soul-personality, who will receive the Prana according to the four modes of assimilation in the functioning of the inner worlds they define.

a) The Emotional World: This is the nature and quality of the emotions experienced by a human being, which first polarize in the *pranic breath* at this level. A lack of self-control – in emotions and and in pulses often translates to bad breathing, and a contraction of the whole sphere governed by the third chakra will weaken not only certain "pranic wavelengths" but will also be a generator of energy waste.

b) The Affective World: This is, of course, feelings. It was self-evident, for the ancient therapists, that shifts in the elevation of these feelings affected the pranic wave in the same way as emotions, with similar implications but directed primarily toward the subtle counterpart of the cardiovascular system. There is as well a "cardiac prana"—namely, a pranic layer, which governs more particularly the balance of feelings, potentially impacting the heart muscle.

c) The Mental World: Analogously to the two previous worlds, our cerebral world, our personal "intellectual cosmos," are more or less powered by the quality of specific prana. This affects the whole of the cerebral cortex and acts on the state of, as well as the quantity of, neurons. So this "pranic coat" directly impacts the quality of the reception of information, all of what we say our brain receives from our consciousness. It also affects the speed of our receiving capacity.

It should be noted that, contrary to modern science, the Ancients, on whom we rely here, did not place what we call "intelligence" or "mental faculties" in the brain. What we now deem the whole brain was simply, for them, a bridge between consciousness (located in the higher spheres of being) and the physical vehicle. The brain is not just an organ within the skull. It is the seat of the soul, and the true "Intelligence" center.

For the Ancients, one of the functions of the Prana was to properly maintain a person through mental, respiratory, and spiritual hygiene. Should it be pointed out that the nature of the thoughts of a human being makes him or her more or less receptive to this third layer of the pranic wave?

d) The Supra-Mental World: We finally approach here the more unknown function of the Prana, the fourth, which affects the supra-mental universe. It is not surprising that this is still embryonic in most of us. Its outbreak, which is starting to be felt exponentially, naturally leads us to address it. Any therapist should be informed about it.

The supra-mental sphere is defined by a superior state of consciousness, allowing for the harmonious union (and efficiency within the incarnation) of the cardiac intelligence and the superior cerebral intelligence. This sphere is a state of perception located beyond analytical understanding and the "classic" loving approach to everything. This state expresses a stage of realization for the being, who takes off from the world of phenomena. It opens the door, allowing gradually for the perception of what is hiding behind the Illusion.

The world of the supra-mental—or of *noüs*, if we prefer the Gnostic term—was defined by Christ as the world of Tekla, in reference to the name He gave to the eighth chakra germinating for some of His followers. When we interpret all this today, it seems obvious that the four layers of the pranic wave only fulfill their luminous and nutritive functions for those of us who sense mounting in them the effects of Tekla. How does one access the reception of such a quality of Prana? The answer is in cultivated wisdom, in love and purity—in other words, beyond any recipe.

At an aura reading, the flowering of Tekla is manifested by the appearance of a luminous sphere that is a white-silvery color about one foot, seven inches above the body. This sphere, which appears first like a small soap bubble, expands depending upon the spiritual maturity of the person expressing it. The sphere is in the area of the luminous gushing of the seventh chakra, where it makes us think of a small ball that "dances" in the flow of a water jet.

It goes without saying that the Prana of "supra-mental quality" is currently assimilated by only a small proportion of humanity. The type of therapy presented in this book, above its healing function, is meant to help readers "work" toward the direction of such assimilation. Its study and practice require indeed a constant and demanding marriage between an understanding of the laws governing the subtle biology of life and a "cardiac" comprehension of the Divine Principle active in every being. The good assimilation of the conveyed potential of this fourth expression of the Prana provides a knowledge of the other that exceeds rational analysis translatable by words. It is sacred spontaneity.

This particular dimension of the Prana brings us now to the Akasha, since it proceeds directly. In the same way we saw the Prana flowing in the Ether in variable proportions, we must understand that the Akasha also penetrates the Prana.

There is no more a waterproof barrier between the Ether, the Prana, and the Akasha than between the Physical Body, the Soul, and the Spirit. These dimensions are extensions of each other.

We can say their active proportions vary according to different persons and also according to locations, since the Essenians as well as the Egyptians saw our Earth as a living being, in the full sense of the term, with organs, systems, and chakras with multiple functions.

4) The Akasha

Its Energy is generated by the *Spirit of the Divine*. This is a kind of emanation or the most direct Divine "secretion" we can benefit from. In other words, we can say that the Akasha is the *Essence of the Light* in the most clear state. It is the absolute spiritual matrix of everything, the Presence of the One who circulates in the Universe of the Universes.

The Unity that the Akasha expresses can be broken down into four forms of expression, and, at the end of an expansion of consciousness, the chance to enter it is given to us. The immersion at the heart of the intimacy of the Akasha allows us to realize that it is "woven" of pearl wires that intersect in apparently random ways, although in reality it is very organized. These wires create kinds of "spiderwebs" in three dimensions that generate true and beautiful rosettes. These shaped roses are not fixed but rather in a state of constant change, exactly like if they were translating the most sacred of the mathematical dances.

At each intersection of these wires or filaments is born a kind of spark or golden light outflow with pink shades. If the eyes of the soul can approach one of them, it will be understood that it is indeed a real cell with a nucleus, at the heart of which is a seal with an imprint evoking "an archetypal letter." In our present historical cycle, the Egyptians seem to have been the first ones to discover this "secret," which illustrates that all that is conscious or not is intimately connected to the Divine.

Sharing this information here is not so the mental capability of the therapist can be nourished in excess but rather so that his or her supra-mental dimension, which is supposed to settle in him or her, can perceive the profound meaning and scope. We must reiterate the fact that the Akasha is the Divine in a pure state, and, from that, the goal of the Esseno-Egyptian Therapeutic Tradition is to bring the ones who adopt it closer to the Absolute Energy of the Akasha.

All communicate and we are all connected (...) Nobody suffers without the whole Earth also experiencing the pain.[6]

In reality, this Tradition invites us to work with a Force that could be named Luna-Solar or Solar-Lunar, as it appeals for the marriage of the Prana and the Akasha. It is asked to go beyond the classic use of the Energy of the Earth-Moon (Blue and

Yellow), which joins mainly the Ether and the Prana in variable proportions. Regarding the thaumartuges, these exceptional beings heal radically with the simple radiance of their loving presence. The Ancient Ones believed they were spontaneously working with the Energy of the Sun-Earth. They were aware of the Wave of Life flowing without barrier, from the causal world to the primal root of the physical world, which, in today's world, we call the cell. This is how we can understand the principle of the *healing of cellular memories*. The healing power of the miracles, performers, or thaumartuges expresses itself in the color violet, an association of blue and red. Red is the representative color of the Akasha.

If you received a guest to your table, you do your best to honor him. This implies you are doing some work inside your home to make the invitation a success. Well, my friends, understand when you wish to receive the celestial Forces – whatever you name it – this implies that you have cleaned your house and you have set up the table.[7]

5) Knowing How to Concentrate the Energy of Healing

Beyond knowledge, where the data may seem to us to be somewhat technical or at least theoretical, the therapist apprentice is always dealing with another question: How does one call on and concentrate the Energy of Healing? Actually, we can understand to some degree what the Force is about when we channel it toward an unwell person. Discovering the way to invite and then to condense it can be a personal challenge to meet.

Here are two practices that can be of help. It is always good to practice them regularly.

1. A First Preparation Before Practice: The Sphere of Light
The priests and monks of the Tradition, which we refer to, developed two very simple practices whose main purpose was to expand the nadis and the plexus. For the therapist, these are the ways and main joints through which the Wave of Healing is called to circulate.

   a) The first practice is to sit comfortably—hands on the knees, palms facing up—and close your eyes. Find a silent moment for centering.

b) Once this is done, join the hands very slowly, ensuring that each hand in its hollow is forming one half of a sphere. When the hands come together very closely, one becomes well aware that each, in its movement, will have "harvested" a certain potential of the Energy of Life.

Once the two hands are shaped like a cup, with only a few centimeters separating the hands, focus now on the spherical space created between them. One quickly notices that this space is composed of a subtle "matter," which is slightly flexible. This presence is palpable in your palms, giving you a very clear sensation of holding a true "Bowl of Light" in your hands. Hold it a moment to "densify" your perception. Then you can tint this bowl green, violet, or white.

c) The next phase of the exercise involves choosing one hand (it doesn't matter which) and placing your energetic sphere in it. Your two hands, still shaped like a cup, will now move away from each other and land slowly on your knees, palms up. One of them carries, as described, the sphere of energy.

d) The second-to-last stage of the practice now requires some visualization. The idea is to "bounce" the bowl of energy from one hand to the other, back and forth, with harmony and joy, exactly like playing a game. Each hand strives to feel the presence of the Bowl of Light each time it reaches a palm. With this movement, its energetic mass is strengthened. The bowl of energy grows a little and tends to densify.

e) Finally, when you feel it's time, bring the two hands and the luminous sphere to your chest, in effect offering yourself the Energy of Healing that has been condensed. Let the force penetrate easily, and then thank the Divine for Its action in and through you.

b) A Second Preparation Before Practice: The Solar Circulation
This preparation is perfectly complementary to the previous one. It also requires visualization, or at least a capacity to "sense."

a) The starting position is identical the first exercise: sitting with each hand palm up, one on each knee, eyes closed, with an inner attitude of relaxation and receptivity.

b) Call for a Presence of Light to descend from the top of your skull. This manifests in the form of a luminous ray that you invite to go down slowly to your cardiac chakra. Then, pause to feel it in the center of your chest. Call in peace and joy.

c) You now move the ray of light to your left arm. Let its energy of life go from top to bottom until it reaches the end of your fingers, moving toward your right hand.

d) The fingers of your right hand then instantly receive the flow of energy, which goes from the bottom to the top of your arm until it finally joins the cardiac chakra. It has come full circle.

e) Repeat this circulating Movement of the Light effortlessly as long as you need to. You are creating an energetic, circulating movement clockwise, which has the effect of dilating the nadis of your arms, hands, and rib cage.

With a little practice, you will notice that this movement operates more quickly by itself. What matters is not its speed but rather its fluidity and then harmony, through which the full Circle of Light will accomplish its work of boosting, cleaning, and soothing the circuits called to work in priority toward the therapeutic touch.

We call this practice the Solar Circulation. It is one of the most important factors in the practice of these therapies.

**Each woman and each man is a priest by themselves.
At the moment of their birth (...),
each one is capable not only of perceiving
the Light without intermediaries,
but you can also invite it to stay in your heart
without the permission of anyone.
Being a priest means being to open to the Divine,
to receiving It at your table, and to reflecting
It around one's self a thousand ways.[8]**

**Each one of us is a Temple that is dying
to forget that It is one.**

**Invite, then, the Divine to take over all
of Its place within You,**

**not just a little bit...completely,
totally, absolutely.**[9]

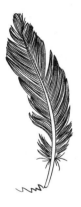

FOURTH PART

The Notion of the Sacred

THE ATTITUDE OF THE THERAPIST

We have said before that the practice of the Esseno-Egyptian therapies would not be what it is today if there was not, at its origin, above all a state of spirit, implying a state of being. This state of mind is simply the sense of the Sacred, meaning the intimate perception that everything originates in the absolute Unity of the Divine, from Its expression, and demands, therefore, respect and love. From there, anything can organize itself. Without this, we miss out on Life.

1) BEHIND THE TECHNIQUE, THE ATTITUDE

A priori, crossing the threshold of a therapeutic approach such as ours, everyone agrees on this basic principle: The quality and expertise of a therapist rely on his or her attitude—attitude toward the sick, of course, but above all the therapist's attitude facing the Energy that he or she is calling and condensing, with the goal of offering. On this path, the student must become immersed in inviting the Divine into him- or herself. If not, he or she would only be a battery partially charged and would have very little to offer a client. The therapist's expertise would not increase. He or she will be limited to memorization and then the application of a set of techniques, interesting and efficient to a certain point but deprived of their real puissance.

The techniques you will find in this book are not at all recipes. They will not act like an aspirin to fix a stomachache or soothe a headache quickly. The techniques are issued from the depths of Life, and their destiny is to act upon our depths.

Of course, not everybody is a mystic. We are not advocating spending time praying and meditating between two clients in order to maintain closeness to the Divine and ourselves.

Anyone who is called to heal others is first destined to be a man or woman "in the field"—in other words, to respond to many demands in multiple circumstances and having his or her days fully booked.

What is the attitude to be developed for the heart of the therapist to be at the height of the task he or she is engaged in?

It is in the constant research of the Divine Wave continuously present in all and not in the subtle duality that is maintained when we rush into five minutes of silence or five minutes of meditation in the hope of becoming centered. It is then in the progressive installment of a state of spirit that makes that all—absolutely all—by becoming a permanent meditation, namely peaceful and loving with the Presence of Light in every form of Life encountered. It is about an ideal, of course, but an ideal that one should not be scared to prioritize. It can be easier to approach than we think as soon as compassion drives us, not a quest for power.

The Sacred always talks of Itself. It doesn't need us to point to It, comment on It, or prove It. The Sacred is and expresses itself by Its Mere Presence, without the need for flattery from words or sentences. It simply whispers to the soul: "Don't say anymore. Open yourself and listen.[10]

At the heart of this attitude and the communion with the Sacred it involves, humility is inevitable, a virtue sometimes difficult to maintain facing the first encouraging results obtained.

If understood, though, the Esseno-Egyptian therapist realizes that he or she will always be a student, namely "under construction" and thus wondering about the prism of Life that is constantly unfolded.

What to add to this? Letting go, of course. From this kind of relaxation of the will that goes beyond the intention of the one who heals, there is no room for tension, for personal appropriation of promising results, or even for impatience.

If we marry compassion and humility and let go, we achieve a kind of equanimity and a loving transparency, a state of being allowing one to act both horizontally and vertically.

In reality, the personal challenge of the therapist—or rather his or her mission—is to find a meeting point of these two "energetic directions." The consciousness of Aton in Egypt was nothing more than a prefiguration of the Consciousness of the Christ. This is the perfect inner space in which to invite the Essenian and Egyptian therapies.

We have already stated that in our Universe, three great types of Waves of Life exist: the Etheric Wave, the Pranic Wave, and the Akashic Wave. They interpenetrate and meet in order to generate and then support the life of an incarnated being.

From there, we must understand that the state of mind and state of being of the therapist tend to be closer to the Christ Consciousness only during "moments of grace." It is more these three trains of Waves tighten and concentrate until they overlap sometimes.

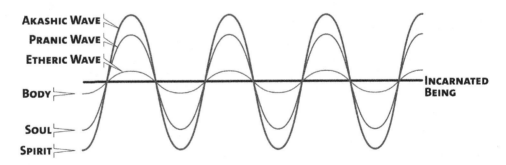

When there is a total overlap of these three Waves and they symbolically draw a sort of cross, what is occurring is most likely what we call "miraculous healing," a consequence of the perfect alignment of all the declinations of the Force of Life. In our approach, there is the need to a call for the Verticality—by the Union with the Divine—simultaneously at the transmission—at the Horizontality—from a compassioned Energy.

One of the keys to approaching this state has not yet been evoked. It is about Trust. It was even named "Abandonment" by the Essenians and Egyptiansthis kind of absolute and sacred letting go, which means something akin to "Lord, I surrender myself to You."

**Never we retain Light within ourselves.
We invite It. We allow It to act.**

**It visits our inner recesses,
sometimes causing trouble,
above all trouble.**

**Then we tell It:
'Dispose of me. You are at home.'**

But never we retain it!

The Ocean doesn't belong to its waves.[11]

2) THE TRIANGULAR RELATION

Such a communion of spirit with the omnipresence of the Sacred leads the therapist inevitably and naturally to extend even more of his or her awareness of what's happening—or should be happening—in the act of healing. In fact, the relationship he or she must maintain with the Divine would be incomplete if not transmitted to the client. Any healing work operates in a triangular manner not only at the physical level but also at the levels of the superior vehicles of consciousness of the being. Work aims toward the healing of a being not only at the physical level but also to those of the superior vehicles. It operates in a triangular manner.

There is not the therapist and the Divine Principle. Neither is there the therapist and the client. Rather, there is the Divine Principle, the therapist, and the client. Such a truth seems obvious when it is expressed; however, we have noticed that it is important to constantly repeat it, as our society is accustomed to operating linearly.

The Essenian teachings of the Krmel already emphasized regularly this kind of chronic disease generated by the duality that makes us think the world is made up of "the others and I." It is indeed a "hereditary disease" at the level of the soul, but it would be wrong to believe that we must inevitably experience it.

Any intelligent relation to Life is necessarily Trinitarian. A binary movement encourages one to mentally "tread water," while a dynamic trinity produces a circulation of energy calling for expansion.

It is not by chance that most great spiritual Traditions lay claim to the Principle of the Trinity.

The drawing of a pyramid from above can illustrate fairly well, albeit in a schematic manner and therefore imperfect, the way that Unity is translated by Three. It allows expression by an Archetype, an Element, a Color, and a Function in the way the Three, which is One calls quite naturally the Four to manifest its existence. The very top of the pyramid represents, for its part, the Unknowable.

With the number Four, we can easily visualize the treatment room of the therapist: a well-grounded place, a room for stability and balance that invites the soul to look up and then rise. This is the temple we have already evoked, a simple space but dedicated by its atmosphere and the suggested athanor that leads the client to rise, letting him- or herself "aspire" to the Above and to thus return to the Divine what he or she has received.[11]

This approach to the Divine Dynamic of Life was part of the database called "secret" communicated to the therapists-priests of Ancient Egypt. We consider it useful to point out here, even though it is already known by some.

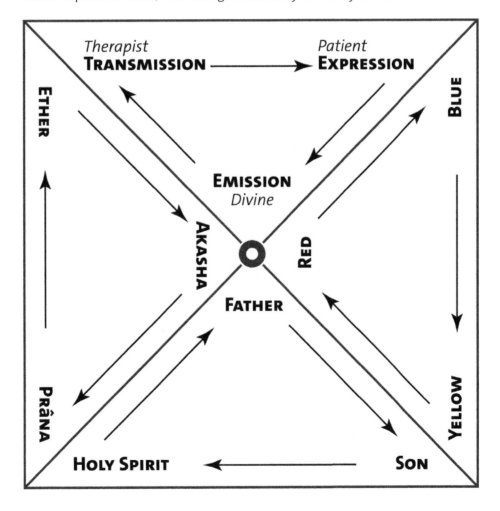

Take refuge in the compassion. It is in this strength you will overcome fear and you will have the perception of what is fair in the eyes of the Divine.[12]

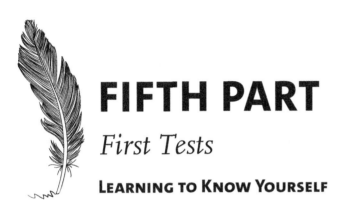

FIFTH PART

First Tests

LEARNING TO KNOW YOURSELF

Before embarking on the practices themselves, it is obvious that a beginner-student must learn to know him or herself in the energetic therapies. We are not talking here of knowledge as to motivations or relatively to internal balance but rather the mastery of his or her perceptive abilities. The following pages have accordingly a goal of helping the beginner-student better identify the "fields of the perceived," which should be explored as soon as we concretely want to take the path that is ours.

Before writing one's first word and then first sentence, each child has to learn the alphabet and how to trace the letters. This is what this is about. At a purely practical level, it is clear that the hands of the therapist are his or her first tools. Therefore, you need a good understanding of your hands and must refine their potential for perception and action. Knowing how to palpate the energy emitted by a body is the basis of all learning in the Essenian and Egyptian therapies. How does one do this? Let us place ourselves in a hypothetical situation.

1) LEARNING THE ETHERIC PALPATION

a) The first thing is to work with a "volunteer-client" who is willing to accept the exercise. The client needs to be in his or her underwear because clothing prevents energy from being released from the body. Direct access to the skin and to the whole physical body is the condition sine qua non for serious and precise work. The use of oils also will subsequently justify this outfit.

b) Your client should be lying down on his or her back or belly. Meanwhile, you are on the client's side—no matter which one—very centered in your body and soul. The Ancients used to put a hand on one wrist or shoulder of the person they were healing, a way to make contact with and install a form of synergy. We strongly advise doing the same today.

c) Once harmony is settled, you stop any physical contact with your client, and you position one of your hands about one meter (39") above the client's body (for instance, in the area of the third Chakra, which is generally easy to detect*). Put there all of your "perceptual consciousness," and then you let your hand go down slowly, vertically, onto your client's body, running your hand with small upward and downward movements to "palpate" the invisible radiance of his or her organism.

---

*Note: *This exercise must be repeated from the top to the bottom of the body by reviewing all the Chakras.*

---

d) At one point, you should feel a kind of small resistance in your hand, indicating a change of "density" of the energy you are looking for when you're palpating. This perception may feel similar to touching soap foam floating on the surface of a bath. Your hand may sense many times such a change of density while going down the body of your client. This will be the sign that you have gone through the privileged sphere from an aura to another.[18] When arriving a few centimeters from the body, the sensation of density should be at its maximum point, a sign that your hand is "engaged" with the etheric reality of the body.

* See map of Nadis p. 29.

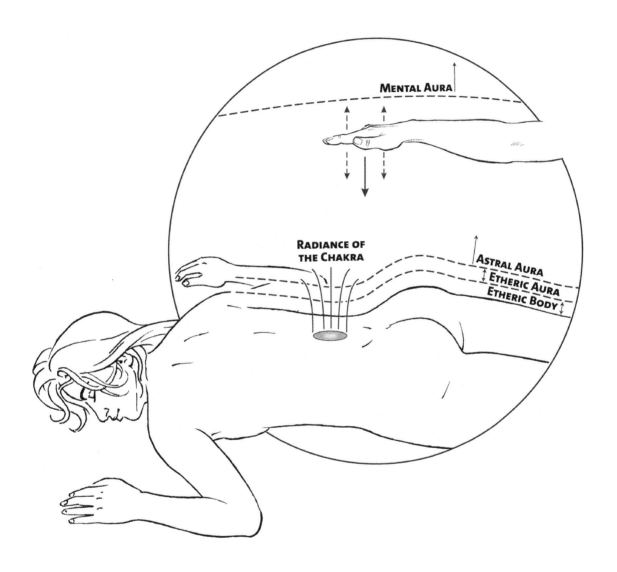

MENTAL AURA

RADIANCE OF
THE CHAKRA

ASTRAL AURA
ETHERIC AURA
ETHERIC BODY

It is crucial to repeat this exercise of approach many times in a confident but neutral way—namely, without aiming for perception at any cost. With practice, your palpation will be able to begin above any Chakra. Although some persons are more sensitive than others, only with practice will a therapist gain a fair and meaningful approach to entering in relation with a subtle organism. The letting go of the therapist, his or her absence of "mental intention," will always be the key to good perception.

2) Emissive Hand or Receptive Hand

During this first learning phase, it is quite possible that you won't feel anything in your attempt at subtle palpation. The reason can be very simple. It may be that you spontaneously used the hand that was less appropriated for this exercise. If we are right-dominant, for example, this does not mean that our most sensitive hand is necessarily the right hand. You must know that we all have two poles within ourselves. One is receptive, and the other is emissive. This translates naturally into our hands, systemizing the pattern of global functioning.

When practicing, some of us clearly have a receptive hand and an emissive hand, while others, relatively numerous, manifest some capacities of reception and emission at the level of the same hand. This is why we are talking more accurately of an active hand for a hand that has both capacities and a support hand for the other hand, which doesn't mean that the other is incapable of emitting a minimum if necessary.

During the practice of palpation described previously, it will be up to everyone to try the exercise by testing once with the right hand and then with the left hand to determine the active hand with his or her own sensitivity. Again, this phase of learning is essential because it conditions and directs all that will enable the therapist to offer a real quality of therapy.

Being attentive, listening to ourselves and to our most subtle perceptions, is an absolute golden rule. Knowing how to trust ourselves without "telling stories" is another thing.

3) Zones of Sensibility

Once you have determined which of your hands is the "active hand," you will need to bring more of your consciousness into it. The goal sought is understanding how it works—that is, to be able to say where exactly it perceives and also where you sense it "wants" to give by emitting the Wave of Healing. For some people, this may be the whole hand, without any particular zone of distinction. For the majority of us, however, precise points more than others keep our attention. We can say that these points are globally three in number:

- *The extremities of the fingers*
- *The palm of the hand*
- *The "secondary Chakra" of the wrist*

Unless the perception of one of these zones spontaneously comes to you during the first tests, you must cliently palpate to determine which of them "answers" better or, in other words, sends you a signal, whatever this signal may be. The question to ask now is this: Once you have determined the active hand, the major zone of sensitivity, does it mean that by this zone of your hand you are going to both feel and emit? The answer is no, not necessarily in any case. It is most likely that your privileged zone of perception or palpation is not the one you will emit the Wave of Healing with. For instance, if you feel the subtle emanations of an organism better at the level of the secondary Chakra of your wrist, you may feel that the Wave of Light chooses to go through your whole hand or by the extremities of your fingers when treating. It is especially true, as we will see, that some Essenian and Egyptian practices encourage therapists to jointly use three fingers (the thumb, the index finger, and the major finger) as "tools of propulsion" for Light. Here again, you have to test them to know your active hand better and to enter into the refinement of its receptive and emissive capacities.

Such tests are not reserved only for beginners because it is not uncommon that the zones of sensibility of a hand move to the other hand over the years.

4) The Nature of the Perceptions

So far, we have talked about "perceptions" or "feelings," but it must be said that these words, though understood globally, are still loaded with a certain vagueness. A little practice in the fundamental learning of subtle palpation will be enough, in fact, for you to ask yourself the following questions: "How do I interpret what I'm feeling? Why do some therapist students not feel the same thing I do?"

The response to these two questions is once again simple: because every human being is unique, with his or her personal story and specificities at his or her own vibrational level, leading to the capture of "life" in a way that is naturally not like that of others. So where some hands perceive a tingling, others feel, for example, heat. Which ones are right, and which ones are wrong? None of them. The message sent by the body of a client is always the same. It is, instead, the nature of the decoder, represented by the therapist, that may vary.

In learning the Essenian and Egyptian therapies, everyone will have to learn to calibrate—in other words, to decode the language of perceptions that is transmitted through his or her hand.

Some schools may tend to systematically codify the signals sent by a subtle organism by asserting, for example, that a sensation of excessive heat means an excess or an engorgement of energy or that tingling translates to an inflammation while a cold sensation suggests an energetic gap. Even if these general landmarks contain some truths, they are still schematics and certainly not applicable as a grid of absolute reference for all therapists.

The famous saying "Know yourself" is the first truth referred to by the

Egyptians and Essenians, each group with their own terms. The notion of calibrating mentioned earlier is, in fact, another basic rule to observe. During your learning experience, the best way to know how a body or, precisely, your hand will translate an energetic ray is by practicing with a person whose health issues you are aware of. It is not required, though, to have a client with a serious health problem in order to calibrate your perceptions. Indigestion, a sprain, temporary liver weakness, or even an intestinal disorder will suffice. You can then build your own referential grid shortly. For example, a sensation of tingling may mean for you a type of dysfunction, while heat or cold is something else.

One thing is certain, however: The perception of a kind of breeze slightly fresh and fluid when approaching the body, the client's dorsal axis, or even an organ indicates for sure good functioning. It is exactly like how the presence of the Harmony of Life circulating rightly can be universally recognized by the same signs! Don't hesitate to repeat the first steps. Their mastery will guarantee the correct interpretation of the "music sheets" you will encounter thereafter.

The key is to be a river by accepting that water is flowing through yourself. [13]

5) Positioning and Seating

We discuss here a point that is much more important than we generally believe. This is about the positioning of the therapist relative to the body of his or her client, who is lying down. In fact, as much as client comfort is paramount, with adequate heat, light, and atmosphere being necessities, so is the comfort of the therapist. The act of healing must in no way be difficult, painful, or generally distressing to hold. If this is the case, it is conceivable that the quality of the treatment will suffer because postural fatigue or muscular discomfort inevitably eats energy and prevents relaxation.

In search of good positioning, two possibilities are the therapist working with the client lying on a massage table or kneeling on the floor on a mat placed for this purpose. The Ancients very much preferred the latter choice. Sitting on a mat or cushion close to the sick person, they favored being in direct contact with the floor— namely, with the telluric force. The energies of Mother Earth were perceived by them as the frame of a cocoon that can do its part in the regeneration of an organism and of a soul in disharmony. They were aware of connecting with this force through the base of the body. The first Chakra is not by chance called the "root." However, this decision implies that after the first approaches for a client, they already knew "in their heads" the total protocol of the proposed treatment. This protocol permitted them to decide their ideal positioning relative to the person to heal: At his left side or right side? To his head or his legs? This doesn't mean that they stayed "nailed" in the same place during the treatment, but the rule was to avoid moving too much. The reason is easily understandable: The less we change places, the more we can maintain the same concentration in the work and the less the client is distracted by movements around him or her.

The choice of a good location will enable the therapist to avoid squirming during arm and hand movements, which will eventually disorganize his or her sitting. An "intelligent" treatment is characterized by a minimum of displacements around the body of the client. This ancient rule of working remains as valid and important nowadays as in the past. The high quality of interiorization and comfort of the client, as well as that of his or her therapist, are the basic but critical conditions to be respected. The problem is less acute in the other case, the one in which the therapist works with a massage table. He or she will be able to move discretely around this table without distracting the client and can avoid squirming or disrupting his or her seat.

Is this to say that this last method is preferable to the previous one? Not necessarily, because it's colder and more technical aspect can influence, from either side, the perception of the Sacred driven by the therapies of Essenian and Egyptian origin. It is therefore up to each therapist to decide in what way he or she prefers to work, knowing that each choice has advantages and inconveniences.

∼

A soul always gathers with its own hands,
with patience, love, and will, one after
another, all flowers that will form,
one day, the bouquet of its radiance.

A being is building himself, in truth,
more than he is built...

A matter of personal decision
because the spark of the Divine expands
only where room is made for It.

All the room! [14]

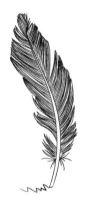

SIXTH PART
The Protocol of Initialization

1) The Good Positioning of the Client

Let's enter into your treatment room, your sacred space, the one you made as a small temple dedicated to the Light and to the service of others. Everything is there: simplicity, warmness, soft lighting, cotton towels, a blanket, cushions, a candle, incense, oils,* and, if desired, peaceful music. Even in the learning phase, it is preferable that all of the elements be set up because the creation of ambiance inviting to internalization promotes the good integration of the teachings.

The righteous learning of our discipline cannot in fact be satisfied with a simulation of the contact with the Sacred. It is about respecting, from the beginning, the good internal attitudes as well as the good external conditions.

Let us now come to your client. What position will you ask him or her to take? Lying down, of course, but which side? On the belly or on the back? The first thing to note is whether the client is at risk of suffering from discomfort. For example, some people may not tolerate being on their belly well. Obviously, this is the case with pregnant women.

Ideally, in the Esseno-Egyptian tradition, the client is first asked to assume a prone position against the floor, head turned to one side, in order to present his or

*See p. 185.

her back to the therapist. As we will see, some elements of this approach protocol for the client justify this starting choice.

In case the prone position is not possible, however, the supine position or even the side position ("three quarters") will be suitable. It is especially important to not be rigid and to respect first of all the comfort of the person receiving the treatment.

Imagine now that your client is lying down in front of you. Are you going to immediately look for the internalization in order to initialize his or her energetic approach? No. Doing so would overlook a point that is very important: the straightness, from head to toe, of the client's body.

With a little attention, you will actually notice that few people lay in a "straight" and harmonious way. Most will not have their legs extending in a straight line from the pelvis and the chest. Consequently, from the start you will be responsible for correcting this misalignment.

To do this, you will place yourself at the feet of your client. Simultaneously take his or her two heels in your hands and lift them up. Then pull the client's two legs softly but firmly toward you so they are correctly set in the axis of the body. This is a simple act but one with great importance for the good circulation of the energies to be treated.

STRETCHING THE FEET

This preparatory phase is called The Stretching. It was considered so obligatory by the ancient therapists that the student who omitted it during an exam would automatically fail.

The Labyrinth existing between the body and the mind is pure fruit of the imagination.

To understand it, to break down the false walls, we must dare to push into it.[3]

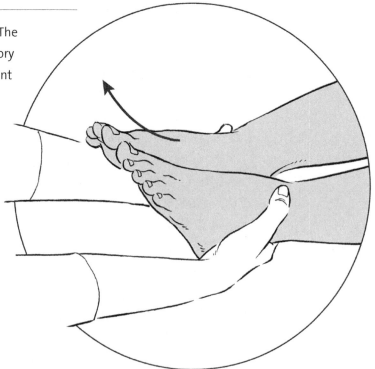

2) THE FIRST ENERGETIC CONTACT

a) Tracking and Palpation of the Median

a) You are finally alongside your client. You have helped with his or her body position, you have chosen the side (at his or her right or left side), you prefer working a priori, and you have internally aligned yourself in order to receive the help of the Divine. Your first move is now to enter into energetic relation not only with the client's body lying in front of you but also with his or her different layers and soul. To do this, you are going to practice what we have previously called "the Etheric Palpation."*

b) You will accomplish this exercise methodically and fluidly, from top to bottom and vice versa, at all the client's levels by lingering particularly in the region of each Chakra. You will obviously be very attentive to all the perceptions, even the ones that seem fleeting. The intended goal is to give you a first impression, the most precise possible of the general state of the organism you are going to treat. What are the areas that hold your attention? How and, at first glance, why?

c) During this exercise of "entry into matter," you are palpating in particular the median axis of the body, *its median*. This can be done simultaneously with your two hands if you feel the need to facilitate your task. The median is the energetic spinal cord of an organism. It is the generated axis by the three major Nadis: the Ida, Pingala, and Sushumna.** Such an axis can be perceived quite easily, like a "pipe" that is quite dense stretching from the head to the tailbone. Its palpation—done most of the time at the level of the emotional aura and the etheric aura—allows generally the re-

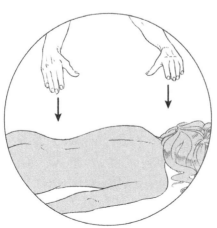

PHASE OF APPROACHING THE MEDIAN

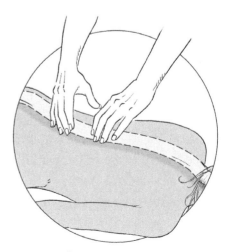

PHASE OF PALPATING
the perception of the median

* See p. 53.
** See p. 31.

finement of what a global palpation has already permitted you to feel. The radiance of the Chakras is then more meaningful.

d) During this practice, you will certainly experience the keen and rising sensation of holding between your hand or both hands the "pipe" of the median, as though it is "something" curved and dense. Your hands will naturally fold into a half-bent shape over it, without tension. In this phase of the exercise, you will also feel perhaps that one of your hands rises up by itself to enter into the vibrational space of such or such Chakra or, on the contrary, that it perceives a kind of energetic void calling it to go down toward the body. Please note that, internally, the upstrokes (voids) and downstrokes (full spots) are always easily interpretable "barometers" that can guide your reflection and, consequently, the nature of what your treatment will be.

In summary:

- Allow yourself all the necessary time to accomplish these first phases of the approaching exercise.
- Note internally your different perceptions when you come in contact with the multiple layers of the body (e.g., impressions of hollowness, outgrowth, windiness, etc.).
- Note precisely as well the points that attract your attention because of the release of their heat, coldness, tingling, etc.
- Do a synthesis of all of it and get a global idea of the "energetic scheme" of your client, a scheme that will not always agree with what the client reported he or she is suffering from.

b) The First Deductions

As much as this energetic, global perception relates to the scheme it suggests, it doesn't have to be something unchangeable and definitive. It is just the first decryption requiring later refinement. Thus, the moment will come when you will internalize differently for a few minutes to establish the complete protocol of the treatment you're proposing. This protocol will consider, of course, the complaints expressed by your client but also what you have perceived of him or her, which may be something the client is not aware of. This will bring you to treat perhaps an area, an organ, a network of Nadis, or a Chakra that—a priori—has nothing or little to do with the symptoms the client is asking your help with. All is connected in an organism. This is a truth to remember.

A reminder: *The Esseno-Egyptian therapies are holistic by nature. They are not looking to treat symptoms by themselves but rather focus on the source(s) of them to understand why there is a malfunction of a system within the inner-workings of the most secret and subtle of the being. Beyond the zones and circuits of suffering, these therapies focus on detecting the impact of possible cellular memories, the schemes of erroneous mental or emotional functioning, as well as affective scars and further traces of a karmic nature.*

Caution: *It is rare that a disease, a specific permanent fragility, or a recurring disorder has its origin only at the etheric-physical level. In the elaboration of your protocol of treatment, you must make sure to not be trapped by the possible complexity of the levels of the being. The ancient therapists-teachers required their students to be connected to the spirit of synthesis.*

In fact, in the same way that an excess of medical drugs, potions, or plants is harmful to an organism, an excess of energetic practices becomes as much. This book offers a number of applicable techniques for various diseases or disorders. You must understand, however, that during your learning experience, these techniques are not to be "stacked" one after another without discernment. The Essenians, like the Egyptians, couldn't imagine the consecutive application of more than three or four healing techniques with the same client.

By "healing techniques," we mean "specific treatments." This term doesn't include what is described in these pages as being "the basic techniques" or "the approaching techniques," which are kind of energetic "entries of matter" applicable immediately to all clients or at least most.

Once well assimilated and with your protocol decided, it will then be up to you, according to the principle already stated, to position yourself ideally beside your client and to offer not only the best of yourself but also and above all the purest of what you are calling to come down onto him or her and on you.

We always end up receiving
the Love we have distributed.
I talk about the true Love,
simple and without calculation,
not of this travesty that we reward
him or her with what they feed
our excuses or serve our purposes,
even unconsciously.[15]

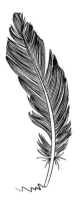

SEVENTH PART
The Basic Techniques

B efore diving into the study and practice of the Esseno-Egyptian therapies themselves, you still have a number of points to assimilate. They are simple gestures or brief technical elements that will come back systematically in most of the described practices in the following pages. It is understood that without a mastery of these elements, it will be in vain to want to go further in this chosen direction.

The gestures you are going to discover are kind of like the ABCs. In terms of the first practices that will follow them and that they must be absolutely assimilated until you achieve fluidity. It will be similar to learning words and how to articulate them. Such words and the nascent sentences you form will be your base as you learn the Essenian and Egyptian therapies. They will constitute an essential database that quickly becomes—as you will notice—a kind of energetic surgery you will practice all the more naturally and precisely, as you will have devoted time to grasp the essence and the logic.

To better understand the meaning of our gestures and their scope, it is necessary, however, to answer two questions: What body do we operate on, and how does the treatment travel from this body?

Unless it can be specifically indicated for certain practices, most of the technical strokes, movements, and "applications of Light" that you will be taught to make will rely on the etheric organism of the client. Does this mean you are not working beyond the first vibrational layer of the being? Not at all! We have already mentioned how well the ancient knowledge we are referring to considered the multidimensionality of the human being and always looked for returning to the source of disharmony. Nevertheless, the Egyptians and Essenians relied initially on the etheric zone of the body because they recognized that it was like the privileged portal facilitating the penetration of other layers in the organism. They found that the etheric body, as a vital relay between the dense and the subtle, transmits the Wave of Healing simultaneously to the "top" as well as to the "bottom." They used the etheric organism like a bridge over the multiple layers of the reality of a being. Of course, they were aware that a bridge may need many "legs" or "arcs" according to what it needs to reunite and unify. In the case of these therapies, the number of "legs" depends inevitably on the intensity of the Luminous Breath emitted by the therapist during his or her practice. You must know that the Wave of Healing, there-fore, travels by "bouncing" from one layer to another in a being, based on the power of the momentum given initially from the "bottom."

1) THE BASIC GESTURES

a) The Union of the Fingers

Each finger of the hand emits naturally its own ray, but we must remember this: The union of the thumb, the index finger, and the middle finger of your active hand will specifically create one of the most precious of your tools. The more you bring your consciousness in it, the more you spark a real beam of energy, which, like a small "laser ray," will be able to act with precision in treating a zone.

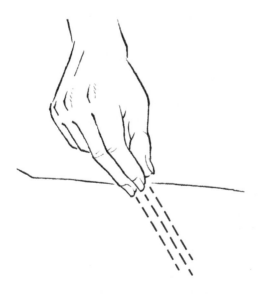

THE UNION OF THE THREE FINGERS: *The ray or the brush. The Ancients associated the thumb with the force of the Uncreated, of the Unknowable; the index to Fairness and the middle finger to the Great Dissolvent, which is Time.*

As a general rule, the luminous beam that springs at the tip of the fin-gers' union projects itself at a distance of ten to fifteen centimeters (three to four inches). In order to test yourself, slowly unify your three fingers and approach a body wherever it is, realizing the fingers indeed emit a healing beam. At a given time when you arrive with your United Three Fingers a certain distance from the skin, you will have the urge to "touch" it with the extremity of your beam. You will know then that you are entered into your "zone of action."

Either you will feel the need to immobilize your beam on the point it touches—a place you have beforehand, of course, determined as a precise point to treat, such as the gallbladder—or you will decide to "sweep" all of an area, similar to using a brush.

If you choose the *light brush*, you will operate it with small, flexible moves, slow and precise, from top to bottom, exactly like painting the skin of your client. With a little practice, you will feel the need, with closed eyes, to tint your light beam while applying it. Don't force it, and don't impose a color either. These will spring up spontaneously. The ones with a real healing power are green, violet, white, and gold. You will likely discover the decongestant power of the emission of such a ray (for instance, on the sinus or even on a vesicle) or its cleaning action. You also will notice that your client will often feel touched physically exactly where you "drop" your ray.

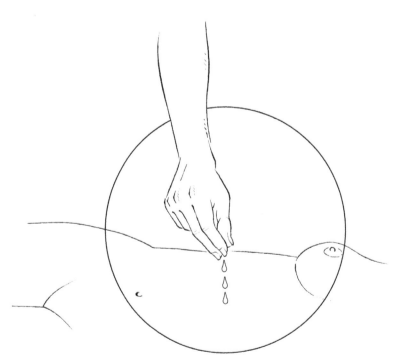

b) The Method of the Dropper

This is about an important variant of the previous technique. You used it "above a precise point" when you felt the necessity to act in a more sustained way on it. The gesture is simple: When you emit your light beam as indicated, you compress your three reunited fingers with small jerking movements, precisely like squeezing a dropper. At the extremities of your fingers, the result will be the spouting of a succession of therapeutic waves more concentrated than the ones emitted by a simple ray. This method can prove to be very effective in the case of pain in a precise zone, particularly at the level of the bladder, the kidneys, and the gallbladder.

c) The Operative Field

We also used the term "energetic surgery." This is in the framework of such work ideally suited to create an "Operative Field" that is vibrationally clean—namely, rid of "energetic slags" (or, in other words, free of waste from the vital body). The implementation of such an Operative Field is extremely simple. It involves the union of the three fingers and their beam being used as a brush.

It consists of creating a grid within the etheric region onto which we project our beam to intervene on this area of the body with the union of the three fingers.

This grid—made, of course, in consciousness and not mechanically—will be a "disinfectant" in so far as it is going to raise the vibrational rate of the zone that benefits from it. This makes it more permeable for the Wave of Healing.

We essentially create an Operative Field where the intervention by "incision"—as described hereafter—is practiced on a major organ.

THE OPERATIVE FIELD

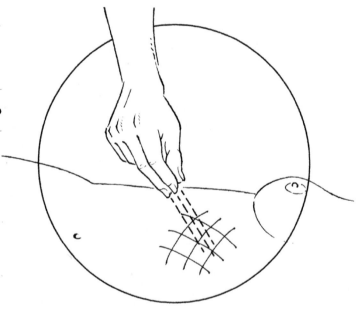

d) The Etheric Incision

This technique is fundamental to the practice of the Esseno-Egyptian therapies. It naturally follows the implementation of the Operative Field just described. You must do your utmost to master it with harmony and flexibility because you will frequently have to use it in the practice of many treatment protocols. Its goal is to enable the Therapeutic Wave you are going to emit to be much more "incisive"—in particular, more powerful in contact with a zone or subtle organ. Its principle relies on the interaction between the blood irrigating the flesh and the etheric counterpart of it.

This technique involves slightly irritating the skin until eventually a small, pink trace appears, so the surface of its etheric counterpart immediately creates a small bulge. You have to learn to feel the presence of this small bulge with the help of your fingers so that you can, without waiting, grasp and form, from its surface, the lips of a "subtle wound."

Here are the details of how to proceed once you've determined the zone you're going to intervene in:

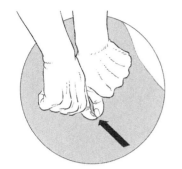

Figure 1

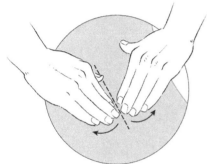

Figure 2

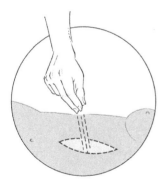

Figure 3

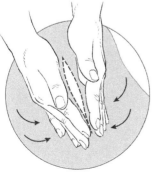

Figure 4

a) Move your right and left hands together so the nails of your thumbs end up against each other.

b) With the help of the extremities of your two nails thus joined, mark a "furrow" directly onto the skin of your client. Your gesture will be repeated from top to bottom, always in the same direction and four or five times in a row, firmly and fairly quickly in order to generate the etheric "bulge" described above. Though it must be energetic, the pressure from the extremities of your thumbs should not be assaulting your client. It's all a matter of finding the right balance in the pressure *(Figure 1)*.

c) Once done, you must strive to feel the etheric bulge that you have provoked with the help of the extremities of your fingers. You are going to "grasp" it with the help of the fingers of your two hands and "separate it in the middle" to create an opening in the etheric body, kind of like a wound with its two lips *(Figure 2)*.

d) At this moment, use the three united fingers of your active hand and penetrate the beam with a light brush at the heart of the opening *(Figure 3)*.

e) Once you have made the necessary energetic deposit, always close the etheric wound with the same consciousness and precision with which you have just worked on it. You may do this with your active hand or both hands *(Figure 4)*.

f) Finally, smooth the etheric zone you have operated on with ample and flexible movements, with one hand or both, from top to bottom.

If the closing of an etheric wound is not done consciously, there will inevitably be an energetic leak at the level where the subtle organism was operated on, a leak similar to one that happens sometimes following a real surgery that does not go well. **Important:** *It goes without saying that we will never practice an Etheric Incision at the level of the heart or the brain, on a fracture, inflamed area, or on a recent scar.*

---

e) The Etheric Extraction

The principle of this intervention suggests extracting momentarily from the etheric body the counterpart of an organ to inundate with Light. This practice refers us to the third stage of the technique of the Etheric Incision—namely, at the moment where an opening on the vital body has just been practiced *(Figure 3 Etheric Incision)*.

a) Instead of unifying your three fingers to classically spring a beam, you are going to open your active hand and place it above the practiced opening parallel to it (and, obviously, in its etheric "zone of sensibility").

b) Once you have established subtle contact with the opened zone, with the help of the palm of your hand making small movements from top to bottom and bottom to top, you are going to "magnetize" the organ that you want to treat, which is necessarily in the hollow of the incised area.

As strange as it may seem, this phenomenon of magnetization is generated easily by the intention emitted by the therapist. So you would apply yourself to the void within you, to visualize and to feel the etheric couterpart detach itself gently and progressively from the body of your client and come to "stick" under the palm of your hand (Figure 1).

c) When you are at this stage, you move your second hand to your active hand and hold "in your palms" the extracted organ.

d) Then comes the most beautiful and sweetest moment of your treatment because this is where you are going to emit to the suffering organ all the love and Light you are capable of producing. This is a sacred moment that you must, of course, dedicate the necessary time to *(Figure 2)*.

e) You then finally let the extracted organ reintegrate gently into its place in the etheric body of your client. This is done naturally by moving your hands apart from each other delicately and going with it in its descent until entering in contact with the surface of the skin.

f) The last step is to proceed meticulously to the closing and then smoothing the etheric wound as described in the previous exercise.

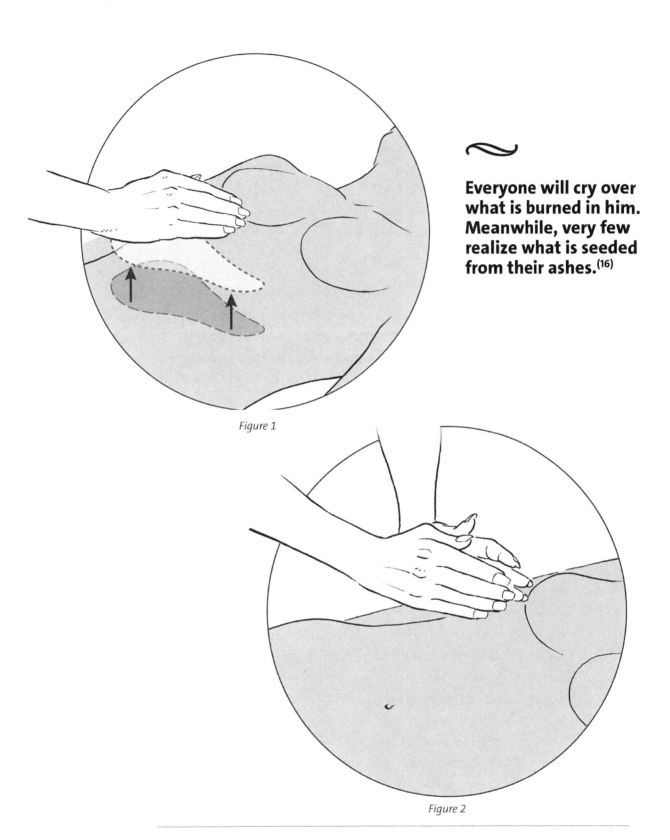

Figure 1

**Everyone will cry over
what is burned in him.
Meanwhile, very few
realize what is seeded
from their ashes.**[16]

Figure 2

Important: *As previously stated, never practice an etheric extraction at the level
of the heart or the brain, on a fracture, inflammed area, or a recent scar.*

f) The Detachment of the Astral Arm

This practice requires a very particular respect for the client and a capacity for important internalization from the therapist. We use it in cases of chronic disorders, recurring problems, or issues that have been buried deeply for a long time. For the therapist, the principle involves extracting the astral arm from his or her physical arm and letting it slide down to a precise area of the body of the client. The mastery of this exercise is not the result of a "technique" in the basic sense of the word but rather an inner attitude that is the fruit of letting go of the mind.

a) At first, place your active hand on the body of the client, slightly above the area to be treated.

b) Simultaneously, place all your consciousness in this hand and your arm until they feel particularly alive. It is possible at this stage that you will perceive an unusual heat or freshness. At a certain point, according to your ability to let go, you will be surprised to find that you no longer "physically" feel your arm and your hand.

c) It will then be time to let "something" release through the extremities of your fingers, like a glove that slips off by itself. This "something" will be the astral counterpart of your hand and your arm. It is going to naturally sink into the subtle organism of your client and will "adopt" the vibrational rate. You will follow it internally, very harmoniously, until you feel it in contact with the suffering area. This sensation can be very precise and may be perceived by your client.

d) Then let your hand more than ever act as Light. It may be that its feels spontaneously the need to "smooth" an encountered organ or remove kinds of scales. Don't intervene with your will.

e) If you experience a sensation of your "full" will taking over you, this will be the sign that your astral hand and arm should be recalled "within yourself." Do this without any physical movement. Both the hand and arm will reintegrate into their flesh support easily with gentleness.

f) After a moment of "communion," observe a little silence, and don't forget to thank the Divine.

Important:
Once again, we never practice this exercise at the level of the heart or the brain, on a fracture, inflammed area, or a recent scar.

g) The Scanner of the Consciousness

This technique is not used for healing purposes but to get information. It enables the therapist to visualize the areas of disorders of a body in its wholeness with a certain precision. So it is a great, useful tool for those who have some difficulty reading auras.[12]

It also offers a complement of information that is very interesting regarding the Etheric Palpation of the body. The Egyptians and Essenians, of course, didn't know about the concept of a scanner. When we choose this term, it is because it makes sense nowadays. They named this technique "the method of the rug." You will easily understand why.

a) Place yourself exactly at the head of your client, who is in a supine position. Press your forehead lightly against the client's forehead, with delicacy and without any uncomfortable pressure.

b) In the continuity of this movement, you gently apply the palms of your hands to the top of your client's shoulders in order to have your fingers lying on the secondary Chakra of each one (in other words, to the anchoring point of the two clavicles). The word "clavicle," which means "little key" in Latin, has real significance because the secondary Chakra of each shoulder plays an important regulatory role for the big vertical and transverse Nadis, from which the subtle organism is irrigated.*

c) You then close your eyes to internalize. At the heart of your internalization, you precisely apply yourself "in review" of the body of your client, from head to toe, exactly like the sweeping beam of a scanner. You will be attentive to each point and each area your psychic scanner encounters difficulties. These points or areas will indicate to you the energetic blockages, disharmonies, or sufferings.

They will be precious indicators. If you experience some difficulty implementing this kind of psychic scanner, then choose, per our illustration, the method of the rug to unroll internally on or in your client. It can provide the same types of indications.

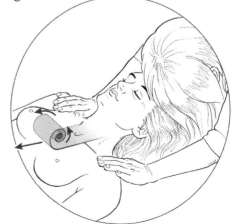

*See p. 29.

2) THE FIRST PRACTICES

By "first practices," we mean here the first real curative exercises through which the Essenian and Egyptian therapy practitioners start a treatment, either in their continuity or partially, depending on the deductions at the time of the initial approach with a client. They are, in their wholeness, relaxing practices because of their process of encouraging flow within the subtle organism enabling it to be fully receptive to the entire protocol of the treatment.

* See the map of the Nadis on p. 29.

a) The Serpentine

Your client is in a prone position (on his or her belly). This stroke is done on the client's back, in contact with the skin. This action can start any treatment, without any reservation. It aims to energetically clean the organism by working on some big Nadis* that intersect in the area. It also has a peaceful effect. If your client is very tense, this treatment can also be done in the supine position so that both sides benefit.

The practice of this exercise is simple; however, we must be attentive to learning it well so as to not reverse the precise strokes. The therapist must make them fluid with natural and comfortable movements. Both hands must slide smoothly.

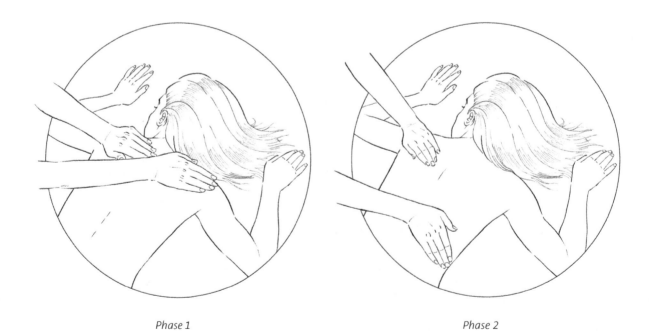

Phase 1   Phase 2

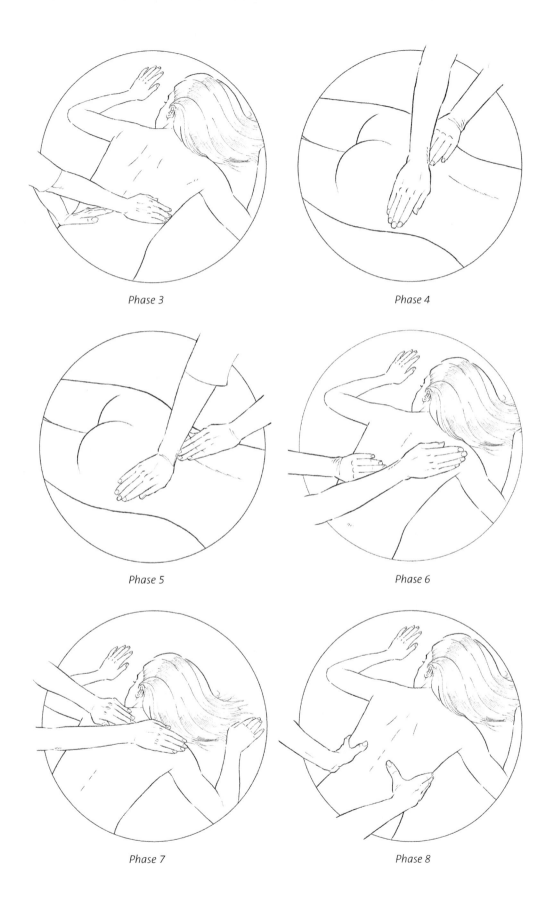

Phase 3

Phase 4

Phase 5

Phase 6

Phase 7

Phase 8

b) Ida and Pingala

The function of this exercise is to create fluidity in the energetic flow circulating along the dorsal axis. This exercise is also practiced on the entirety of the back of the client. While completing the relaxing work of the serpentine, it consolidates the good distribution of the moon-solar Force through the median. It facilitates the plugging of possible energetic leaks along the two major Nadis (the Ida and Pingala).* For some people, the practice of this exercise may seem difficult because it requires the autonomy of both hands acting simultaneously with precise and different small movements.

*See p. 31.

Your client is still lying on his or her belly.

a) Position yourself on the left side of your client at the level of his or her left hip. Face the top of the client's body. Place the extremities of your two thumbs directly onto his or her skin at the top right of the spine. Your left thumb will move up and down and down and up, while your left hand moves slowly down to the bottom of the body along the axis of the spine. Simultaneously, your right thumb will draw a series of lemniscates on the skin of your client, while your right hand goes down slowly to the base of his or her body in the same rhythm and in parallel to the left. Stop at the sacred vertebra.

b) Position yourself on the right side of your client, facing his or her right hip. Your body is situated at the right side of his or her chest. Again, place the extremities of both thumbs in the same direction as in Phase 1, except this time on the left side of the spine from the sacrum. The movements of your thumbs and hands will be exactly the same as described in Phase 1. The only difference is that they will go up from the base of the body to the dorsal vertebra.

Practice these movements over and over until you achieve perfect fluidity and the absolute autonomy of both of your hands. To repeat, you can work first on the movements of your left thumb and then the more refined movements of your right thumb. When each of your thumbs has mastered these movements, you will synchronize both thumbs to obtain a harmonious practice of this exercise.

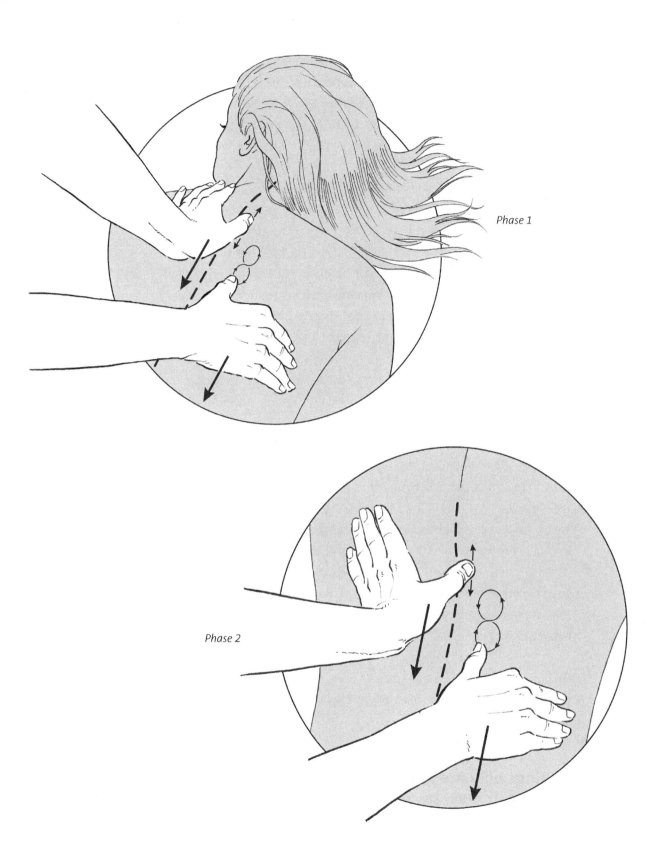

Phase 1

Phase 2

c) The Alignment of the Subtle Bodies

This exercise, also practiced on the back of the client, allows for a great centering of the etheric, astral, and mental bodies. It indeed happens that these bodies are not correctly "fitted together." So if the client mentions being unable to concentrate, sleeping difficulties, and other small symptoms, there is often an atypical, translating desynchronization of his or her subtle bodies.

This is a simple and efficient technique that can facilitate an aura reading when we wish to read in depth.

---

a) Pause your support hand between the first and second Chakras of your client (in other words, between the tailbone and the sacrum). Your support hand stays there for the totality of the treatment. Simultaneously, place your active hand at the top of the client's head, in contact with the seventh Chakra *(Figure 1)*.

b) While your support hand remains in the same place, move your active hand to the sixth Chakra of your client, who is in a prone position with his or her head turned to the side *(Figure 2)*.

c) With your support hand remaining in the same place, move your active hand to the fifth Chakra, behind side of the throat (Figure 3).

d) Your active hand should next land delicately on the dorsal vertebrae at the level of the fourth Chakra. Still, the support hand is not moving *(Figure 4)*.

e) Then the active hand slides to the third Chakra, approximatively to the level of the kidneys of your client. Your support hand will remain still between his or her tailbone and sacrum *(Figure 5)*.

f) Finally, while slightly pivoting yourself, place both hands in an enveloping way at the midpoint of the back of your client *(Figure 6)*.

The beginnings only are powerful because they are just beginnings. It must be with the Breath, the One who operates the metamorphosis of the depth.[23]

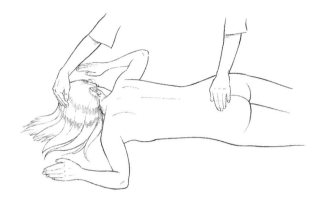

Figure 1

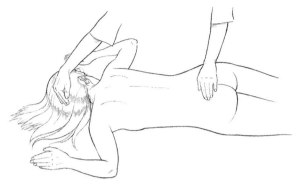

Figure 2

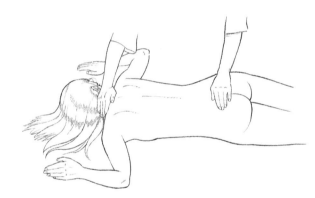

Figure 3

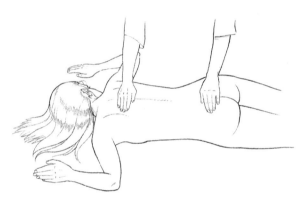

Figure 4

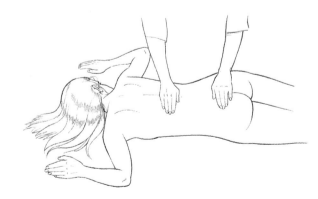

Figure 5

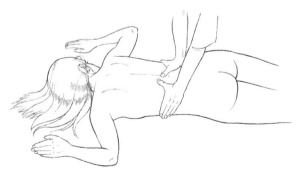

Figure 6

d) The Diagonals

This time, your client is lying on his or her back (the supine position), as this treatment will be applied to the chest. The work is indeed centered on the two major Nadis intersecting the rib cage in the manner of a pair of shoulder straps that meet at the level of the heart Chakra.

This method is extremely interesting, as it facilitates the liberation of painful cellular memories, mainly ones linked to a difficult relationship with society or life itself.

We can use it to calm, for example, people affected by agoraphobia. However, like the serpentine and Ida and Pingala, we advise using it during the initializing protocol because it always plays a liberating role by facilitating the expression and relaxation of the often moral or spiritual suffering of the client. It is not uncommon, for that matter, for it to elicit some tears.

During the practice of this therapy, you will notice that you may be led, with your hands placed directly on the skin, to draw a big X. Make sure that the top of the corners of the X correspond to the two secondary Chakras of the shoulders and its two bases with the two secondary Chakras of the last two floating ribs of your client. Each position will be held for a thirty-second minimum and—this goes without saying—in full consciousness so a large deposit of Light can be made.

You will notice here, as with the preceding first practices of "The Serpentine" and "Ida and Pingala," we ignore the notion of an "active hand" and "supporting hand." When necessary to respect the active hand rule, it will be precise in the treatment.

We imagine that the Soul is located at the heights of the being, but (...) it is always at the deepest of its valleys, indeed in its caves, that we must look for.[25]

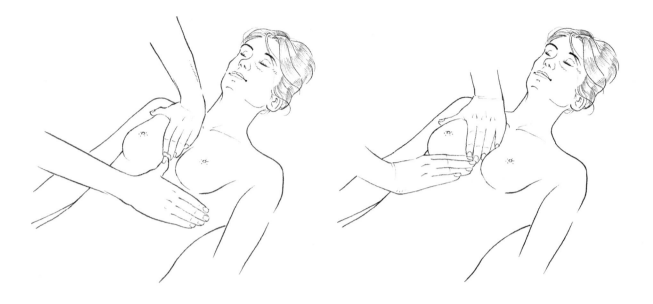

Figure 1   Figure 2

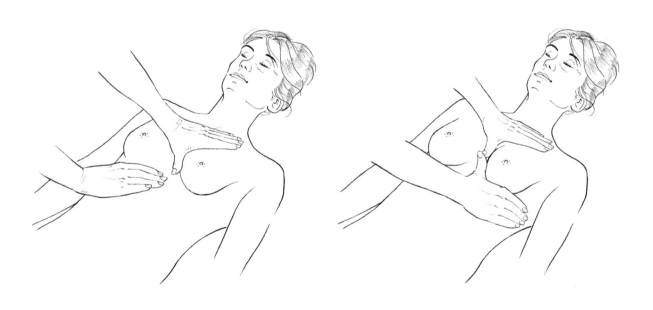

Figure 3   Figure 4

e) The Method of the Umbrella: Balancing the Chakras

This is another fundamental practice that needs to be mastered perfectly. Though appearing very simple, it requires precision, rigor, slow motions, and flexibility. The Ancient Ones used it mostly on the front side of the body; however, it can be applied as well to the back of a client. Its function is to rebalance a Chakra, whichever it may be, except the seventh Chakra, the coronal, and obviously the eighth Chakra, still embryonic, located "outside of the body." The notion of "rebalancing" implies that you don't have to worry whether the (closed or dilated) Chakra you have chosen to heal contains any dysfunction in an organ or other disorders. According to the expression, too closed or too dilated. This means that The Method of the Umbrella is first of all harmonious. It is based on the pure intelligence of the Chakra in its capacity to auto-regulate. So this method intervenes as a supporter or booster of its capacity. Not constrained by the very delicate "mechanism" of a Chakra, it can thus be widely and regularly practiced on a subtle organism.

Here's how to practice this method:

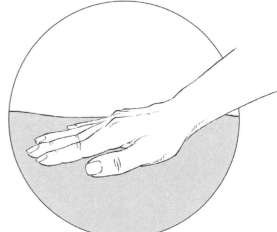

Figure 1

a) First, precisely locate the Chakra to heal. Then lay your active hand flat at the heart of its zone of radiance *(Figure 1)*.

b) With a slow inspiration, close your fingers while lifting your hand gently, exactly like you're closing an umbrella or a parasol *(Figure 2)*.

c) With your fingers still together and while your inspiration is still deepening, let your hand rise about fifteen centimeters (6 inches), just above the center of the Chakra. Your gesture can end with a spiraling motion, clockwise, done with the extremities of your five united fingers *(Figure 3)*.

d) Release a short breath from your full lungs. Then let your hand move down vertically and quietly on a slow expiration while your fingers spread apart. Allow your hand to lay flat in the exact same spot you started from, at the heart of the Chakra *(Figure 4)*.

Figure 2

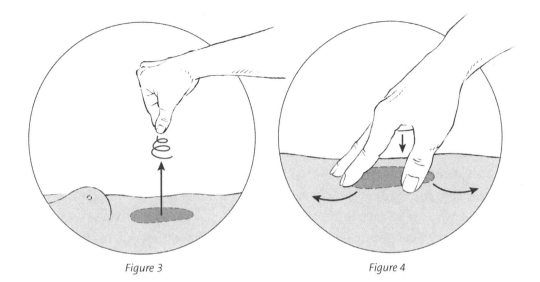

Figure 3   *Figure 4*

e) Once you've regained the position, release another short breath—this time from empty lungs—before redoing the exercise.

To summarize simply, this essential practice can be performed like this:

- Hand flat on the Chakra.
- With inspiration, close the hand like an "umbrella" during the ascending movement.
- Short apnea from your full lungs.
- Lower the hand toward the body and simultaneously redeploy the "umbrella" while breathing out.
- Short apnea, this time from empty lungs.

The sequence of these movements can be repeated five to six times in a row at least (peacefully) and obviously not mechanically. The therapist must learn to feel, here as everywhere, the moment when the "work" turns out to be correctly accomplished.

General Comment: *Each time you open your hand in deployment or retraction when in contact with the physical body or in its subtle space, make sure that your fingers are glued together, without tension of course. This prevents any loss of energy. This note also applies to all of the exercises.*

Know that when a hand is flat on a body, it always avoids scattering its healing power. The ancient therapists noticed that the beneficial treatment of an area is initiated by the placement of an active hand with a number of "luminous seeds." These seeds are born from points of impact on a body area. They grow and between each other form luminous filaments. This intensity restores health. In other words, a hand laid flat with fingers together works by "infiltration" in the sense that it creates a whole vibration without any dispersion.

---

f) The Parallels

This method is often associated with the one concerning the alignment of the subtle bodies. It complements its effects when a client expresses obvious exhaustion. Contrary to the practice of aligning the subtle bodies, though, its action is primarily limited to a cleaning of the etheric body by the "scouring" of two of its main axes of Prana circulation.* The Essenians and Egyptians named the two major Nadis that travel the body from top to bottom and from the right to left side "parallels." Each parallel starts its run at the level of the second Chakra of the shoulder and goes down along the body, ending up behind the heel, with some of its ramifications extending to the foot. Along its path, it will cross—by meeting other Nadis—some important energetic points, mostly the last floating rib, the iliac crest, the fold of the groin, the inner thigh at its half-height, the popliteal fossa, and the inner side of the calf (at half-height as well).

The work of the parallels is easy to apply:

  a) First, without considering the polarity of your hands, place one hand on the secondary Chakra of the shoulder and the other hand behind the knee, at the popliteal fossa *(Landmark 1 – Phase 1)*.

  b) Once you have placed your hands as described above, you will circulate a flow of Light, infiltrating first the top of your skull, going through your heart to your left hand, and continuing then to your right hand and passing by the body of your client, finally reaching your heart again. Continue this to generate a clockwise movement of companionable energy. As a reminder, this movement is called "Solar Circulation"** (Landmark 2 – Phase 1).

  c) In the second phase, bring your hand that was placed on the shoulder of your client to the bottom of his or her rib cage. At the same time, move your other hand from the popliteal fossa to the iliac crest. This second phase is completed using Solar Circulation as well *(Landmarks 3 & 4 – Phase 2). Obviously, you will need to apply these two phases to each of the two big parallels, meaning each side of the body.*

A second method for working the parallels existed, mainly done by the Egyptians. It involved making an important Etheric Incision along each of the parallels and applying the method of the three fingers by using their laser as a brush.*** Practically, this last method is not as easy to apply, even if its efficiency is as noteworthy as the previous one.

* *See the graphic on p. 29.*
** *See p. 29.*
*** *See p. 66 and 67.*

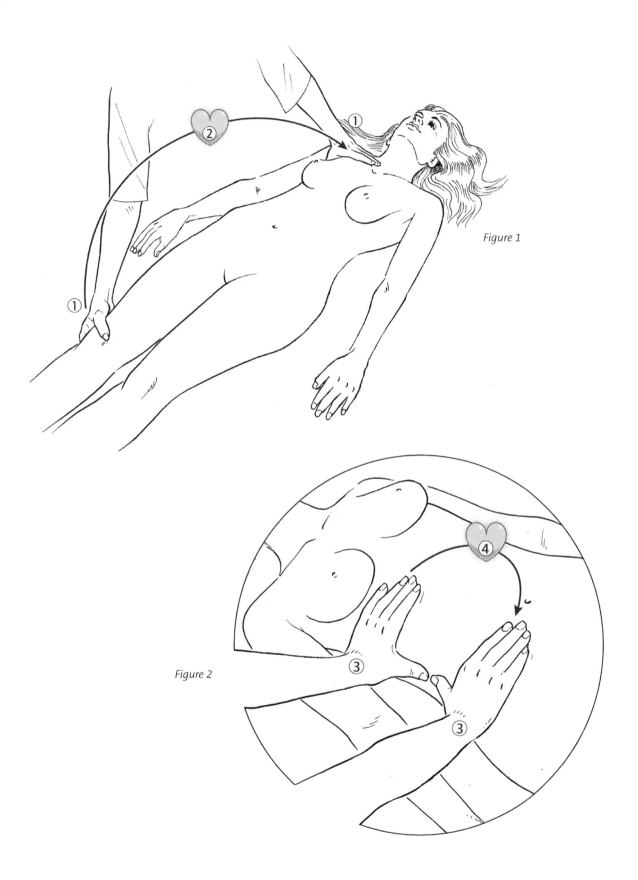

Figure 1

Figure 2

g) The Stream

This healing method is performed on the client's front side. Like the diagonals, it is not uncommon that it brings with it some emotional waves. You will be aware of the precise area of the body or Chakra that will eventually trigger an emotional response or perhaps physical discomfort. The facial expressions of your client will also be very revealing.

In the energy therapies, practitioners often discover that most people who reach out to them are demonstrably emotional and tense. In a subtle therapy, the purpose is not simply to treat a physical problem but to touch the dimension of the soul as well. With rare exceptions, emotions and tensions generally don't present good conditions for fair and deep work. It is preferable to overcome them.

The therapy of the stream is designed well to remedy this by promoting an emotional cleanup of the client—in other words, to work in the direction of relieving him or her. Its impact is thus emotional and mental, although it relies on the dense and etheric reality of the body by allowing the evacuation of certain recalcitrant "slags."

Here is how to proceed:

a) Start by placing your active hand at the level of the pubis bone of your client, fingers oriented to the top of the body.

b) Go up very slowly with your active hand from the bottom to the top of the body to reach the laryngeal Chakra. The principle is simple: Everything fits in these lightweight, "wavy" movements imprinted by your hand moving up along the median of the body. You will notice that these small undulations are easier to make if the palm of your hand is in direct contact with the skin of your client. It slides better this way *(Figure 1)*.

c) During your "ascent," pause briefly at the level of each Chakra so as to perform a slight circulatory movement—clockwise—very slowly with your flat palm.

d) When close to the Chakra of the throat, don't perform this circulatory movement. Instead, simply press the totality of your hand just under the area. Bring your supporting hand perpendicular to the extremities of the fingers of your active hand to draw the letter T *(Figure 2)*.

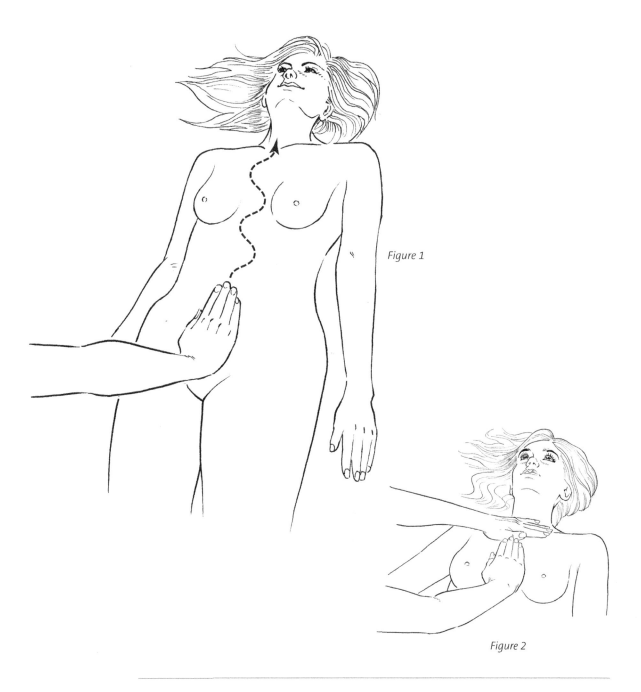

Figure 1

Figure 2

This application of your two hands under and on the laryngeal Chakra should be the gentlest possible because many energetic nodes are concentrated in this part of the body, which is in connection with a very sensitive "part of the soul." Your touch will therefore be lightweight and attentive because it can bring out unexpected sufferings, especially if the client is having some difficulties expressing his or her feelings. Ideally, the gesture is accompanied by a wave of sustained compassion.

3) Some Practices and Additional Data

In addition to these basic techniques, some additional data can help to facilitate and enrich your practice.

a) The Connection: The Gesture of the "Harvest"

This is a very simple gesture performed at the beginning or during a healing session if the client describes feeling "off-centered." The technical gesture is basic but very efficient. It consists of bringing the active hand up vertically, during three to four

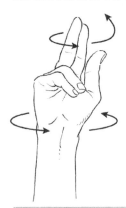

seconds, and imprinting with a clockwise rotating motion. By executing this motion with consciousness and using specifically the thumb, the index finger, and the middle finger like an antenna, we can generate a luminous vortex rich in Prana and Akasha. Such a vortex greatly helps the therapist in his or her function as a "channel" during the triangular relationship already mentioned. And it is obvious that this gesture must be sustained with an adequate state of mind—in other words, with a true call to the Divine.

Connection *Make this gesture as brief and discrete as possible in order to avoid any possible theatrical effect. Accomplished naturally with ease, respect, and love, it doesn't attract attention but touches simply the True.*

---

b) The Luni-Solar Star

During treatments long ago, the Essenian therapists were sometimes challenged by the energetic fragility of a body area or an organ but failed to understand the possible cause. When such a case presented itself, they then used the method of the luni-solar star. With this method, the therapist draws in a single stroke in the Ether above the suffering area a star with eight branches, without any hesitation, eight consecutive times. This subtle drawing was designed to connect the therapist to one of the Archetypes of the Principle of Regeneration and to offer strength to the fragile region of the organism of the sick person. This Archetype is always active. Today, we can use this method when the need arises or as a complement to a session to empower a treatment.

The luni-solar star method corresponds indeed to the Ishtar planet, Venus. It is an ancient contribution that the Sphere of Consciousness issued from this world bequeathed to our humanity a very long time ago.[13] Another method, Egyptian, consists of drawing in the same way the key of life—in other words, the "Ankh"[14] sign of the Egyptians.

c) The Touch and Language of the Skin

We have spoken almost exclusively so far of the different inherent energetic layers of the human body as they appear in physical reality. However, we should not deduce that the Egyptians and Essenians turned away from it under the pretext that the physical body is the "last link" of the manifestation of the being. Although the Essenians, as mentioned, were more distant toward the physical body than the Egyptians, their therapists didn't neglect it. Whatever the body may be, it must be maintained as a temple, where "above and below" meet, share, and become an expression on Earth just as it is in Heaven. For the Ancient Ones, touching the skin of a sick person produced a talkative effect. They had to learn not to remain deaf.

Thousands of years later, this truth has not changed. This is why beyond the Immaterial in the classical sense, you are taking care for what translates invariably to the physical body of your client. Global body temperature; sweat; dry, moist, and tight areas; very warm or "frozen" parts; even trembling all mean something.

Everyone talks about cardiac intelligence as you pass from simple empathy to compassion. There is no need for a reference grid then. Hence, the importance of the respected and loving touch of the shoulder or wrist of your client, already recommended during "first contact," and also the "first practices." We also must be conscious of the fact that the touch by itself, beyond the techniques we use, can sometimes play a major compassionate role, as many people are living alone or are remotely isolated, far from the liberating force of a hand coming to land on them. All is in the delicacy of this gesture, the intelligence of it, and the consideration with which it is imbued.[15]

Like all souls whose wounds hurt, yours will heal only by ceasing to look at where it hurts; in all truth, I assure you, no healing happens by the rejection of a world, of a time, even by forgetting an offense. Healing is achieved by donation. Donation removes the victim from the mire of the discharges and punishments eternally engendering each other. Donation restores the being as he is within himself, face to the Eternal. He is Health, he is Peace.[(18)]

Spirit is so vast that It looks for Itself through the Soul, and the Soul doesn't know what to do if it could not rely on the body. It is through the body that It finds Its way to Spirit. However, the destination is not Spirit, but the Path itself. Because, in truth, the Path doesn't go indefinitely, but it is a place, a unique point at the center of the Heart.[19]

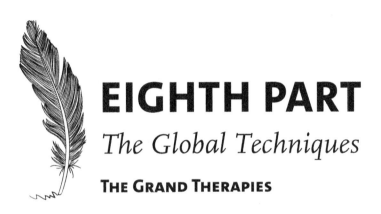

EIGHTH PART

The Global Techniques

THE GRAND THERAPIES

So here we are now hard at work. The techniques that we offer you to discover as a set are often named *The Grand Therapies*. They are global techniques, which one or few elements are somehow the frame of most healing protocols. You will also come to understand, the "technical set" could be the backdrop to other sets more specialized, thereafter named "specific techniques".

Obviously by studying them, you will try to understand the inner logic. "Why such movement or not? Why this order?" If your mind easily understands some gestures or sequences, others will escape from your analysis. To that, the Ancient Ones's response was that the "bodies of the Soul" have a logic that will always elude a good part of ours. It would be vain to try to micro-analyze any technique for the sake of comforting a mechanism of the brain.

1) The resynchronization of the Soul and the Body

This treatment was conceived to help people with scattered energies and symptoms of difficulty concentrating, sudden fatigue, and also slight dizziness. These symptoms generally reflect oscillations between the mental, astral and physical bodies. Without really talking about the "displacement" of the subtle bodies, they appear fluctuating. This treatment is a fast realigning especially useful for active persons.

> a) First put in resonance the second and seven chakras
>   *(Figure p. 95 – Landmark 1)* page will change in the English version.

The resonance is to place simultaneously your hands in two areas of the body and apply the "Solar Circulation". As a reminder see p. 44-45.

> b) Use the method of harmonization of the Umbrella at the cardiac chakra
>   *(Landmark 2).*
>
> c) Massage clockwise – for example with your thumbs – the two secondary chakras of the shoulders *(Landmark 3).*
>
> d) Do likewise for the two secondary chakras of the last floating ribs *(Landmark 4).*
>
> e) Finally repeat this stroke to the secondary chakras of both iliac crests *(Landmark 5).*

Note: For this "mechanical" action, you can act at the same time the left and right side of the body – namely simultaneously with your thumbs of your hands – or treat one side and then the other side.

> f) Finish by a very sweet and loving revitalization of the soles of the feet as illustrated.

Suggested oils (always dilute): "Chakra 1" and "Chakra 7", 'Fusion", "Refocusing", Rose of Damascus Essential Oil.

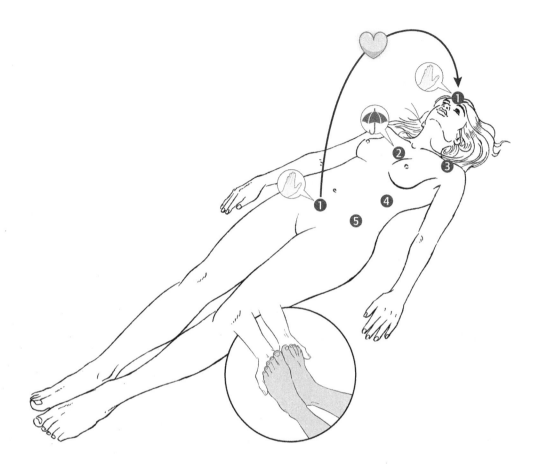

RESYNCHRONIZATION SOUL AND BODY IMAGE
Gestures associated with benchmarks 3, 4 and 5 are also applied to the right side.

Believing with confidence is very beautiful, being aware after having tasted is very interesting, but knowing for finally inviting the silence within is even greater.[20]

2) The grand fatigue

As indicated, this treatment aims to curb persistent exhaustion and fatigue.

a) Make a big Etheric Incision on all the whole height of the body, namely from the pubis to the throat. As the method describes, you will create big etheric lips on the whole abdomen and thorax.
(Figure 1 and 3 – Landmark 1)

b) With The Method of the Dropper you offer the greatest pearls of Light you are capable to the second chakra of your client.
(Figure 2 and 3 - Landmark 2)

c) Do likewise to the third chakra *(Figure 3 – Landmark 3).*

d) Repeat on the fourth chakra *(Figure 3 –Landmark 4).*

e) Do it finally to the laryngeal chakra *(Figure 3 – Landmark 5).*

f) Apply the method of the three fingers brush from top to bottom and bottom to top on the whole incision *(Figure 4).*

g) Close with precision and consciousness the entire etheric opening that you created on the body, then finish by smoothing *(Figure 5).*

Suggested oils (always dilute): "Vitality", "Heart", Spruce Hemlock Essential Oil and Officinal Lavender Essential Oil.

Only Love who planted the seed deserves the title of Greatness, because in it there is already earth, water, wind and sun, the whole tree with its fruits and its oil, all this in promise and abundance, because this is in the light of the look, in the sweetness of the hand, and in what it is hiding behind all of this that there is the sourdough of the Universe. Only this is great".[21]

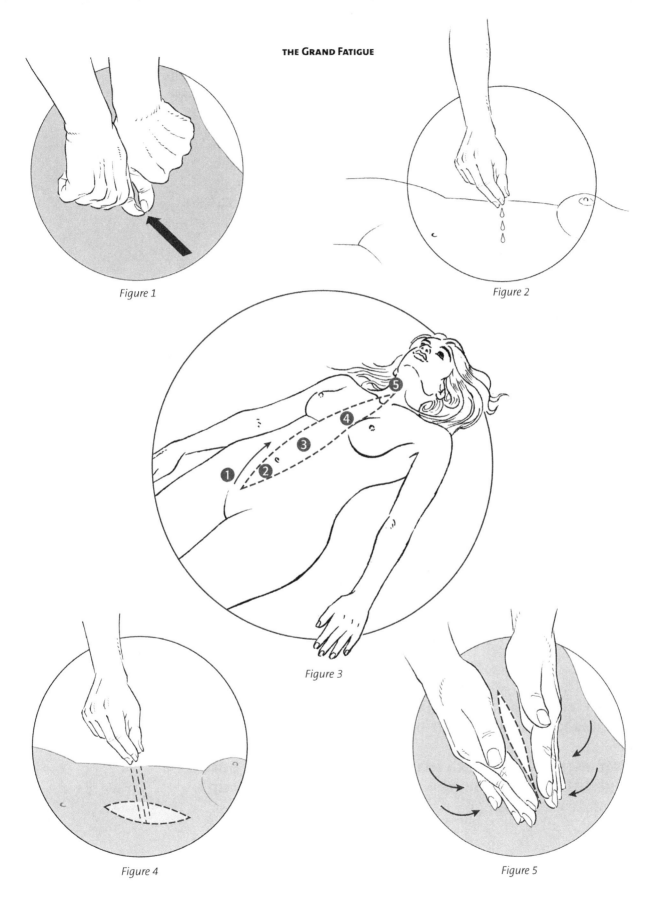

Figure 1

Figure 2

Figure 3

Figure 4

Figure 5

3) THE ENERGETIC LEAKAGES OF THE SHOULDERS.

This treatment can be performed in addition to the one entitled The Grand Fatigue.

It is indeed very common that a very tired person shows significant energetic leakages at the secondary chakras of the shoulders as well a porosity of the Nadis that connect them. This fragility often leads to devitalize the whole ribcage.

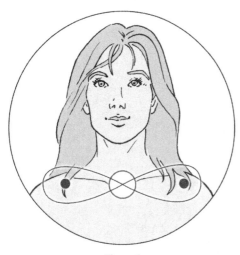

Figure 1
ENERGETIC LEAKAGES OF THE SHOULDERS

a) With your active hand, unify the secondary chakras of the shoulders by a slow, precise and harmonious stroke drawing a lemniscaste. The central point of this massage movement is located in the area of the laryngeal chakra. Repeat this gesture consciously seven to eight times in a row or more according to your perception *(Figure 1)*.

b) Follow your treatment by a sustained imposition of your hands in T. This gesture will go "fixing" the luminous deposit that you offer to your client *(Figure 2)*.

c) Ideally practice a reading of the median and the subtle bodies by palpation in order to ensure the good energetic stability of the treated area.

Suggested oils (always dilute): "Vitality", "Heart", "Repairing Balm", Spruce Hemlock Essential Oil and Officinal Lavender Essential Oil.

There are magic or sacred moments in our lives where an unshakable and superior Puissance uses us as a path.

It makes us feel a truth that we are not always dignified but distances us from the Void and makes us grow up despite everything.[22]

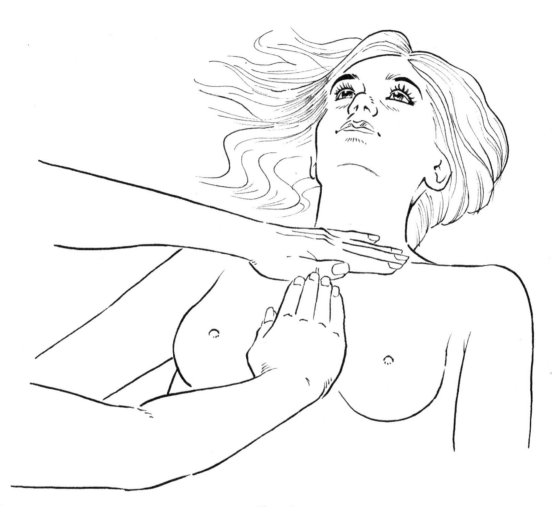

Figure 2
CONTINUED IMPOSITION OF HANDS IN T

4) The states of shock

This treatment holds a place apart in so far as it is used in emergency cases, physical or psychological shocks. This means that it doesn't require any initial protocol of approach described in these previous pages. It is designed to be done rapidly. We can even use it in the case of fainting. However, it must say that this treatment is not necessarily "pleasant' for a suffering person to receive due to some painful pressure points to be done on the body.

The therapist will particularly be cautious to the reactions of his client and find a "moderate" way to address these pressure points.

a) With the thumb of your active hand start massaging clockwise the sensitive point located under the left collarbone (closed to the middle) at about ten centimeters (4") to the right of the thymus. Learn how to find this point. This little massage – energetic without excess – solicits the vital forces and prevents possible fainting *(Figure 1 – Landmark 1)*.

b) Still with your thumb, slightly massage clockwise the secondary chakra of the left last floating rib *(Landmark 2)*.

c) With the same thumb, maintaining your pressure on the skin, go up from the point to another point located few centimeters (inches) above the left breast. You will draw a curve passing by the center of the chest. When arriving at the mentioned point – sensitive to pressure – massage it clockwise as well. Repeat this movement three to four times *(Landmark 3)*.

d) Create a resonance – with The Solar Circulation – the sub-chakra of the left shoulder and the one of the right last floating rib. Do the same with the sub-chakra of the right shoulder and the one of the left last floating rib. You have drawn an energetic X on the chest of you client. *(Figure 2 – Landmark 4 and 5)*

e) Harmonize the third chakra (solar plexus) with the "method of the umbrella" *(Landmark 6)*.

f) Harmonize the fourth chakra in the same way *(landmark 7)*.

g) Hold long the soles of his feet with your hands in order to stimulate and facilitate the anchoring of your client.

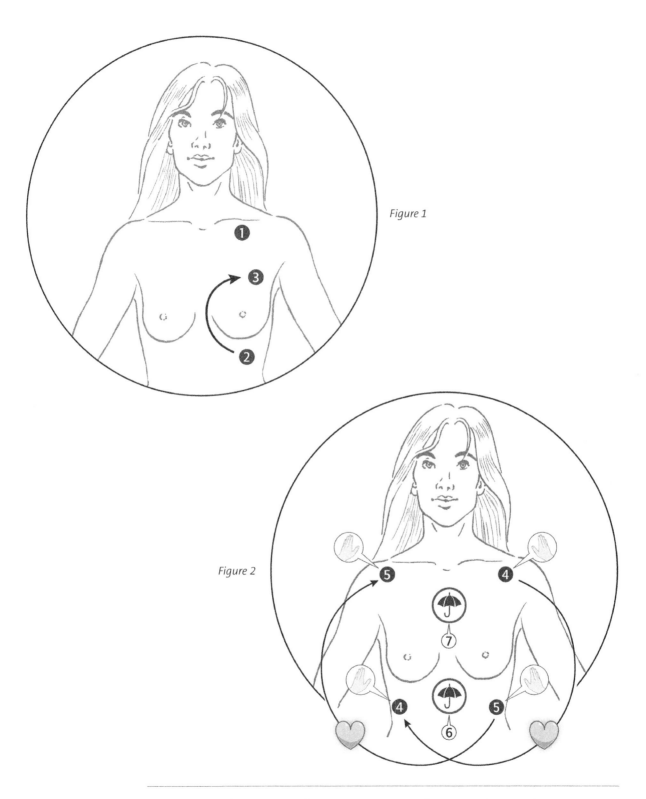

Figure 1

Figure 2

Suggested oils (always dilute): "Emotional balance", "Chakra 1", Rose of Damascus Essential Oil, Myrrh Essential Oil.

5) THE PROFOUND EMOTIONALITY

This treatment is designed to release the energetic aftereffects of an exacerbated emotionality. It helps the client to better master his emotional nature and its succession of disturbances. It is indicated to try to stop deep and persistent emotional disorders. Also it can be used for punctual emotional shocks with the "states of shock" treatment. The therapist will ensure to have a burning candle close by his active hand.

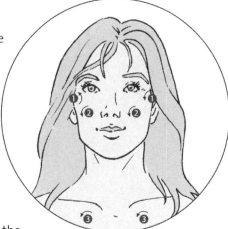

Figure 1

a) Start relaxing your client by massaging counterclockwise the two points located at the superior root of each ear *(Figure 1 – Landmark 1)*.

b) Do likewise with the two other points located in the center of each cheek in direct contact with the superior jaw. These points are always very painful in case of strong emotionality *(Landmark 2)*.

c) Massage in the same way and always counterclockwise the points located under the collarbones, These points are very sensitive as well *(Landmark 3)*.

d) Massage the epigastrium in the same way but with larger and softer movements although still firm. The use of an oil is recommended for this area *(Figure 2 – Landmark 4)*.

e) Apply a strong pressure at the top of the pubis bone for few moments without massaging.

f) Make a long Etheric Incision between the epigastrium and the top of the pubis. After the opening, use the method of the brush with the help of your three fingers. Carefully close the etheric wound and smooth it *(Landmark 6)*.

g) Practice large lemniscates horizontally on the skin from the liver to the spleen with the center located in the area of the third chakra *(Figure 3 – Landmark 7)*.

h) Practice same lemniscates now vertically, namely from the epigastrium to the top of the pubis to include the second chakra. *(Landmark 8)*. The cross that you have just drawn in the abdomen of your client will have the effect to release many stagnant "pranic snags" from the ether of this area.

i) With the help of your active hand, sweep energetically but with fluidity the covered space created by this cross. By sweeping, try to grip between your fingers the polluted etheric mass. With these movements, pass your hand regularly and rapidly above the flame of the candle to purify these harvested snags *(Landmark 9)*.

j) Finally harmonize the third chakra with The Method of the Umbrella *(Landmark 10)*.

Suggested oils (always dilute): "Emotional balance", Petit grain Essential Oil and Chamomile Essential Oil.

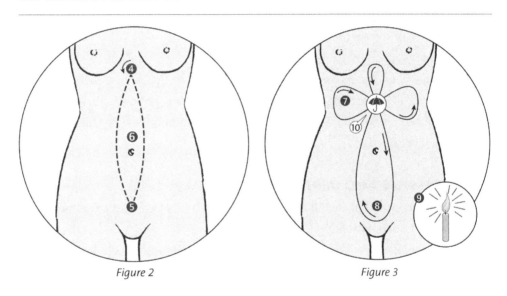

Figure 2   Figure 3

6) A SELF-TREATMENT FOR THE MASTERY OF THE PROFOUND EMOTIONALITY

This treatment is unique in the way that you can advise your client to practice it on himself at will between two meetings with you. It indeed allows a person suffering from acute emotional waves to stem them as much as possible. It is an efficient exercise to practice on ourselves and not on somebody. The process of self-healing is thus somehow different from a therapy applied on someone. Here are the instructions to give your client:

a) Start by placing your left hand on your solar plexus, just above your navel. At the same time, position your right hand at the center of your chest. Remain there for a moment, eyes closed and totally, freely breathing.

b) On the interior screen of your closed eyes visualize the image of a translucent cup that is being filled slowly with a light string of water. When the cup is full, your heart will be also full with a fresh wave.

c) Inspire then expire fully from your lungs: be conscious of expulsing at the same time everything that pollutes your thoughts and your actions. Repeat these inspires-expires slowly, as many times you fell the need. A work of letting go with kindness will happen on your mental crystallizations.

d) Move each of your hands up one degree: the right hand will be placed on the laryngeal chakra, the left hand on the cardiac chakra.

e) Let the silence develop in you and then emit the sound "M" in a sweet but sonorous way. Repeat this sound many times and then fully feel the new form of silence that is installing in you.

f) Finally, join your hands and smile to yourself. At the same time thank the Force of Life for offering the moment to you. Why not dedicate a little prayer from your heart that it is yours, like a leitmotiv when this moment will be renewed?

7) Depression and depressive states

It is well understood that this treatment is not a method of energetic therapy that will fix or heal a depression.

The therapy here is conceived to sustain an interior approach taken by the client himself and is ideally supported by a competent psychotherapist.

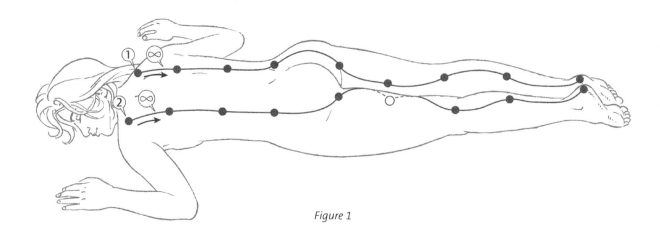

Figure 1

The suggested work aims to clear up the subtle bodies from various types of pollution accumulated that are weakening the whole organism meanwhile the being is getting bogged down in his difficulties. It is a cleansing simultaneously done on the vital, emotional and mental plans so that the client is more receptive to the metamorphosis that his soul requires.

Phase 1: the client is on prone position

a) With the help of an oil, massage by doing small lemniscates on the two great axis that represent the major Nadis that run from the secondary chakras of the shoulders to the heels (*Figure 1– Landmark 1 and 2).*

Phase 2: the client is on supine position

a) The same way you did on the back, massage by doing small lemniscates the two major Nadis that run through the body from the shoulders to the heels. They are the same nadis from the posterior side but they are approached differently *(Figure 2 – Landmark 3 & 4).*

b) Always massage with more pressure by doing lemniscastes and by staying on the nadis of the sole of the feet *(Landmark 5 and 6).*

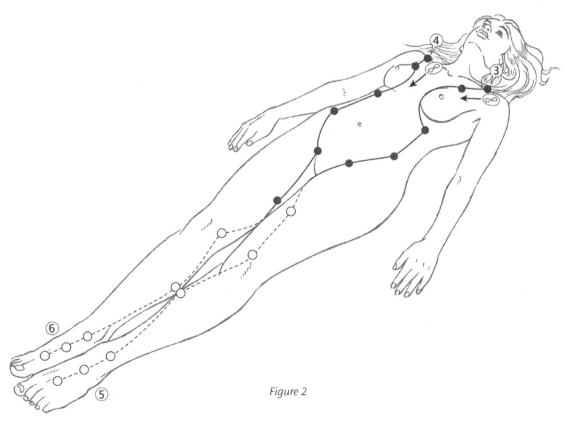

Figure 2

Phase 3

* The silver cord is a true umbilical cord connecting the etheric body to the different vibrational bodies of the soul, astral, mental...

a) Harmonize the second chakra using The Method of the Umbrella (Figure 3 – Landmark 7).

b) Harmonize the third chakra by The Method of the Umbrella. Then, only if you have mastered the technique, detach your astral arm to delicately pet, with your subtle hand, the anchor point of the sliver cord.* It is located in the region of the liver. In the case of a depression, this cord is extremely tight to the point where, in order to breathe, the astral body momentarily leaves the physical body often, creating then a discomfort (Landmark 8).

c) Harmonize the frontal chakra by The Method of the Umbrella, then go down to the laryngeal chakra and harmonize it the same way (Landmark 9 and 10).

d) Lighthly place your both hands on the top of your client's skull and let your heart pray (Landmark 11).

Suggested oils (always dilute): " Chakra 7", "Vitality", "Joy", Jasmine Essential Oil, Olibanum Essential Oil.

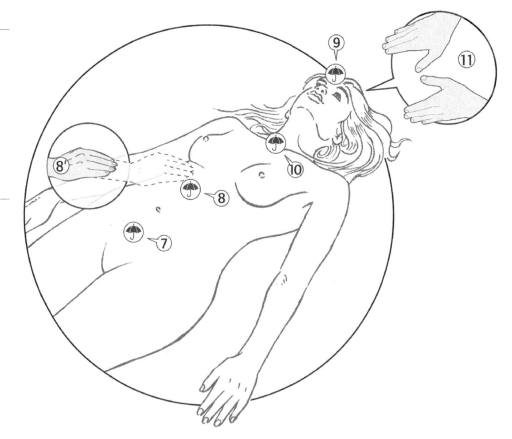

Figure 3

8) The mental crystallizations

The mental crystallizations are energetic waste from the mental body – thoughts of low vibratory rate emitted repeatedly. They are small energetic undefined masses that, by becoming encysted and structured, generate over time what we call "Thoughts-Forms". They pollute the mental body and can disrupt the level of the whole consciousness of a person and affect very subtly his or her balance. Generally, they are from small daily annoying habits.

This treatment aims for dissolving them before they become organized as toxic Thoughts-Forms. It must be known that the treatment can sometimes trigger strong emotions or a sensation of anger with the client, who has to be warned before hand.

This treatment is practiced on the back of the client. The whole dorsal axis has first been coated with an appropriate oil. The strokes to perform by the therapist must be especially mastered and fluid.

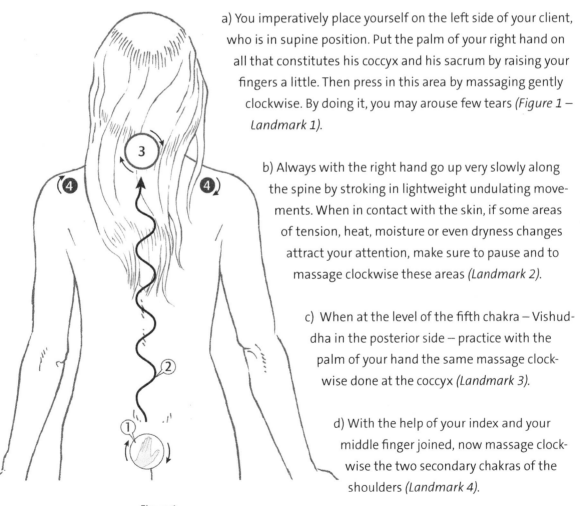

a) You imperatively place yourself on the left side of your client, who is in supine position. Put the palm of your right hand on all that constitutes his coccyx and his sacrum by raising your fingers a little. Then press in this area by massaging gently clockwise. By doing it, you may arouse few tears (Figure 1 – Landmark 1).

b) Always with the right hand go up very slowly along the spine by stroking in lightweight undulating movements. When in contact with the skin, if some areas of tension, heat, moisture or even dryness changes attract your attention, make sure to pause and to massage clockwise these areas (Landmark 2).

c) When at the level of the fifth chakra – Vishuddha in the posterior side – practice with the palm of your hand the same massage clockwise done at the coccyx (Landmark 3).

d) With the help of your index and your middle finger joined, now massage clockwise the two secondary chakras of the shoulders (Landmark 4).

Figure 1

e) Place your left thumb on the secondary chakra located in the slight hollow that can be felt under the protrusion of the left occiput at the base of the skull. This sub-chakra and its right counterpart are "doorways of energetic exit". Massage them counterclockwise to disperse waste accumulations.

Simultaneously your index or thumb of your right hand is placed on the left side of the base of the coccyx to massage it gently and respectfully clockwise, which will create an energetic potential *(Figure 2 – Landmark 5)*.

f) After you are correctly interiorized in the practice of these two inversed yet simultaneous movements, visualize sending a wave of light from the left side of your client's occiput towards the left side of the base of their coccyx *(Landmark 6)*.

g) Now place yourself on the right side of your client and repeat the same movements.
   • Your right thumb massages counterclockwise the base of the right occiput.
   • At the same time, your left index or thumb massages the right side of the base of the coccyx clockwise *(Landmark 7)*.

h) Send a wave of Light from the right base of the coccyx to the right side of the occiput. Internalize well *(Landmark 8)*.

i) Without pressure, and with full compassion, lay your left hand on the whole area of the occiput and simultaneously place your right hand, slighter even, at the top of the skull *(Landmark 9)*.

Some people don't tolerate well that we touch the top of their head: in this case, it is appropriate to remain distant by respect.

Suggested oils (always dilute): "Revealing", "Chakra 6", Lunar water, Spruce Hemlock Essential Oil

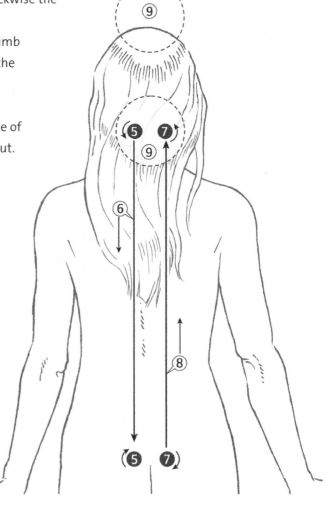

Figure 2

9) THE THOUGHTS-FORMS

The Thoughts-Forms are significant energetic masses that sometimes stay for a long time in the mental aura, and can play an important role at all the levels of the being. There are some who are obviously charged with a constructive potential. The therapist of the Essenian and Egyptian Tradition will focus to detect and defuse those who are compromising the healthy balance of the person.

The Thoughts-Forms treatment is indicated for people who are clearly stifled behind a problem that is not able to be expressed in words because it is encysted in them, which blocks them – consciously or not – meanwhile weakening some functions in their organism that may lead to disease.

a) Your client is in prone position. The first phase of the treatment requires a mechanical intervention to liberate his mental body from accumulated toxins by addressing a number of major points located along of his parallels. This will promote a first "opening up" of the Thoughts-Forms.

We must massage dynamically clockwise with your thumb or index or middle finger of your active hand the following secondary chakras:
- The back of each heel *(Figure 1 – Landmark 1).*
- The back of each calf at mid height of it *(Landmark 2).*
- The popliteal fossa of each knee *(Landmark 3).*
- From the inner face of each leg to its mid-height *(Landmark 4).*
- At the groin folds *(Landmark 5).*
- At the iliac crests *(Landmark 6).*
- Under the last floating ribs *(Landmark 7).*
- At mid-chest level, each side of the sternum *(Landmark 8).*
- At the secondary chakras of the shoulders *(Landmark 9).*

It is important to know each of these points well which, by the way, are sensitive to touch and have a small depression in contact with the skin.

Figure 1

Note*: On the Figure 1 of this treatment as well as all figures of this book, the points noted with a white circle indicate located areas on the opposite face of a limb or a body.*

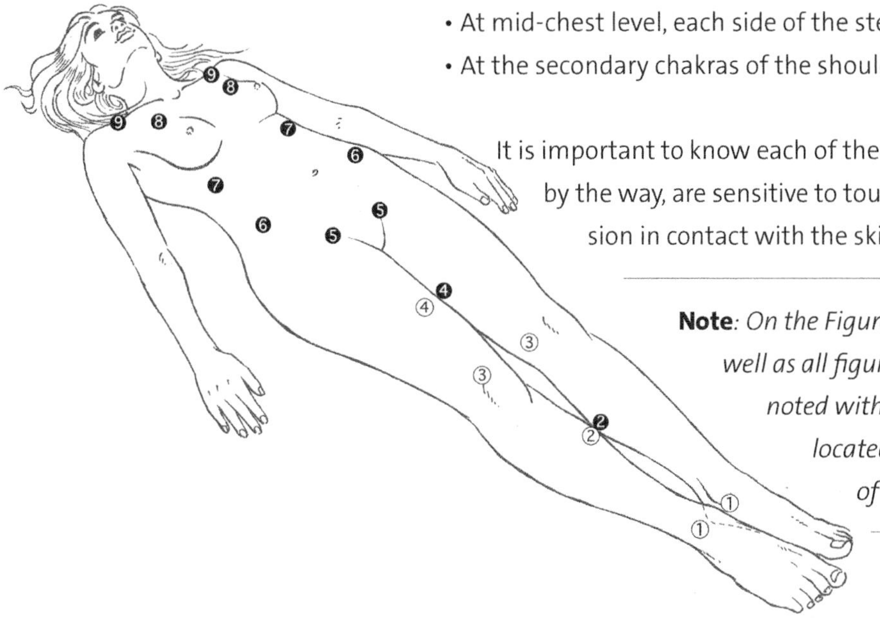

b) Place a small drizzle of oil from the laryngeal chakra (VIshuddha) to the second chakra (Swadhistana). When done, massage in small lemniscates with your two fingers of your active hand from the fifth chakra to the second one. *Caution: This is not a simple massage.* Be conscious of the fact that you are sending a force down from the top to the bottom of the body *(Figure 2 – Landmark 10).*

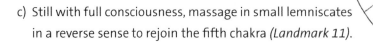

c) Still with full consciousness, massage in small lemniscates in a reverse sense to rejoin the fifth chakra *(Landmark 11).*

Figure 2

d) Simultaneously place your active hand on the second chakra and your supportive hand on the third chakra. Put them in resonance within moments using The Solar Circulation *(Figure 3 – Landmarks 1A and 1S).*

e) Place your supportive hand on the cardiac chakra and, simultaneously as well, your active hand on the third chakra, Manipura. Practice the solar circulation again *(Landmarks 2A and 2S).*

f) Bring your supportive hand up to the laryngeal chakra and your active hand to the cardiac chakra. Practice The Solar Circulation between them one more time *(Landmarks 3A and 3S).*

g) Let your supportive hand placed on the laryngeal chakra and bring down your active hand down to the second chakra. Practice The Solar Circulation on last time.

h) The step before the last phase of this treatment is as important even though it looks like insignificant. You place the body of your client "in sandwich" between your two hands which are positioned on the anterior and posterior faces of the third chakra, active hand above. Meanwhile, breathe clearly for your client to hear your slow and deep breathing. Ask him then to match his breathing to yours for few minutes. Do it with lots of delicacy. This is probably the only time where you need to involve the will of your client during a treatment *(Figure 4).*

i) Place yourself at the head of your client and gently take his cervical vertebre in the palms of your hands. Infuse Light and Love *(Figure 5).*

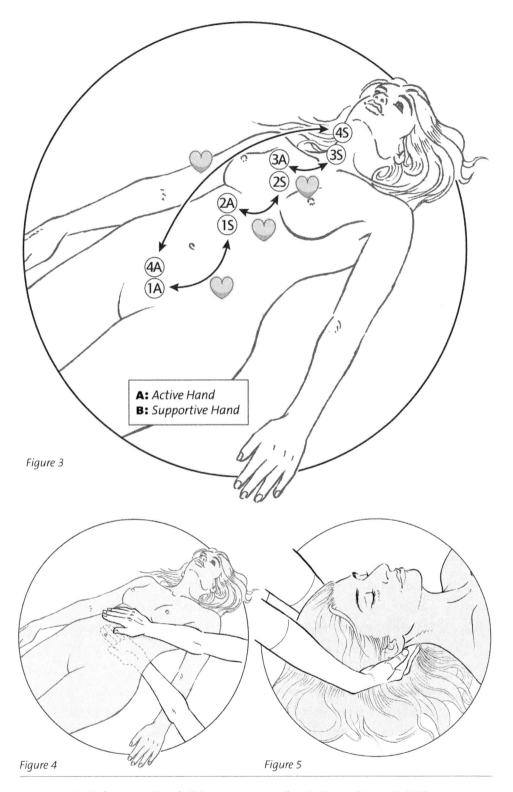

A: *Active Hand*
B: *Supportive Hand*

Figure 3

Figure 4

Figure 5

Suggested oils (always dilute): "Thoughts-Forms" or Spikenard Essential Oil,
Lavandula officinalis Essential Oil.

10) Self-Parasitizing

The Egyptians and Essenians knew this mental attitude of the human being who pushes himself sometimes to self-intoxicate by maintaining attitudes, thoughts and behaviors from a parasitized nature. We are talking about destructuring thoughts that mostly generate fixed ideas, which make them going "in circles" with the same psychological problems that finally attack an organ, an area or a function.

The feelings of guilt and persecution, repetitive attitudes of personal depreciation for example are often from a self-parasitizing that ends up by compromising the functionality of the organism.

The self-parasitizing treatment can be applied complementary to the Thoughts-Forms treatment when the client obviously shows an obsessional feature in his thoughts and behaviors that make them harmful for his own sanity.

This treatment, which must be repeated many weeks, touches the emotional and mental bodies. Ideally, it must be sustained by research permitting the client to realize the trigger of his problem.

a) A burning candle must be imperatively close by you. After spreading a little oil on the dorsal axis on the body of your client, you are placed at his head to delicately hold his neck in the palms of your hands forming a cup *(Figure 1)*.

b) Internalize deeply within yourself and practice the Technique of the Scanner* to determinate one of more areas of energetic blockages. Memorize well what you have perceived and establish priorities within the suffering areas.

c) Place yourself on one side of your client, slide your progressive hand under his neck, and land the other hand on the area of the detected issue. Proceed by order or importance if there are several but not more than three *(Figure 2 – Landmark 1)*.

d) Inhale slowly through your nose and, at the same time, "aspire" by your active hand, the energetic toxic charge of the area over which is placed. It is possible you may feel this charge by a sensation of itch in your palm.

When your lungs are full, exhale through your nose while going quickly with your open hand over the flame of your candle. Begin again immediately the "aspiration" exercise as many times you think it is necessary *(Figure 2 –Landmarks 2 & 3)*.

*See p. 73.

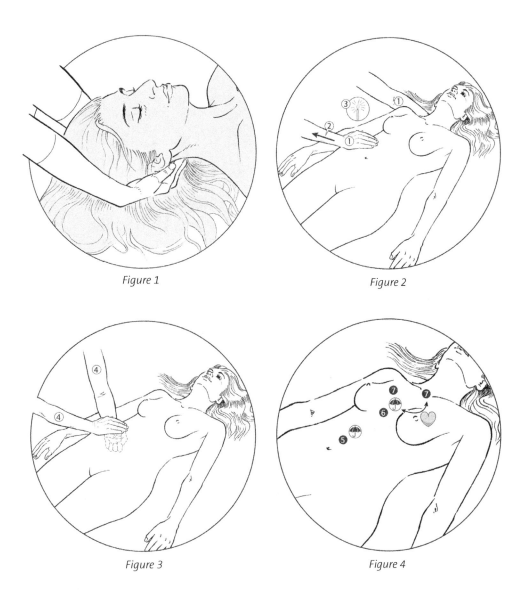

Figure 1

Figure 2

Figure 3

Figure 4

e) Place your supportive hand under the body of your client at the level where one of the additional areas are being treated. Simultaneously your active hand is placed in the front of the body of the treated areas. Call intensely for Light *(Figure 3 – Landmark 4)*.

f) Reharmonize the third chakra, Manipura, then the fourth chakra, Anahata, by The Umbrella Method. Finally bring resonance by The Solar Circulation in the fourth and fifth chakras *(Figure 4 – Landmarks 5,6,7)*.

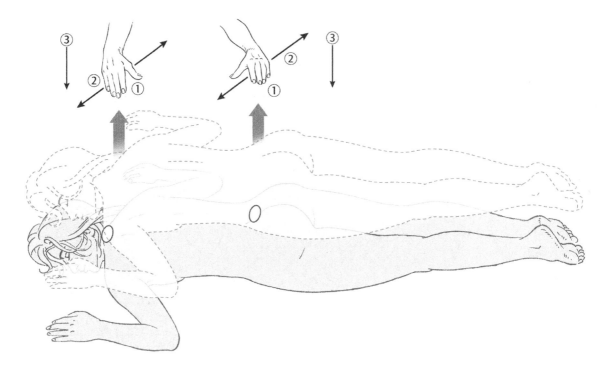

Figure 1

11) MECHANICAL READJUSTMENT OF THE SUBTLE BODIES

It is quite common that the subtle bodies happen to move away from the physical organism. A little emotional shock or a bad wake up can be the causes. The phenomena is then insignificant and absolutely temporal. It can therefore remain if the cause is way deeper, like a violent physical shock, a difficult birth or a badly lived surgery.

The perceived symptoms frequently are: vertigo, nausea, sensations of "walking next to his body" in the awake state, and eventually, headaches.

The Essenians and the Ancient Egyptians had set up a simple and efficient procedure to remedy this typical misalignment of the subtle bodies that are stepped aside from their physical support by a few centimeters or have even become slightly "sideways" compared to it.)

a) You are placed on the side of the lying body of your client and you enter in contact, by palpation, with his etheric organism.
   This contact is established at the level of the second and the fifth chakras. Apply to feel it clearly.

b) Then, magnetize his etheric body by "lifting it up" it by these two points. Remove it from above the physical body about ten to fifteen centimeters. The astral body will follow in the same movement but don't worry about it. Feel the subtle body well as it is coming up within your hands (*Figure 1 – Landmark 1*).

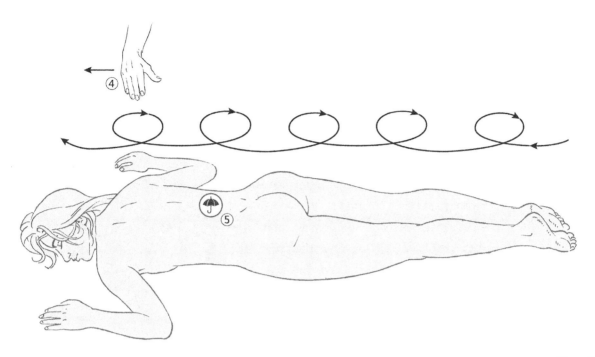

Figure 2

c) Once the subtle organism is removed, make it oscillate two or three times in front and behind, namely towards left then right of the physical body *(Landmark 2)*.

d) Progressively stop your oscillation movement and recenter the etheric body as precisely as possible over the physical body. Then let it down very, very slowly towards the physical body by accompanying with your hands, still placed at the level of the second and fifth chakras *(Figure 3)*.

e) With the help of your active hand, draw a series of ellipses horizontally, from feet to head. These movements are practiced quite fast in the space of the astral aura. It is recommended to repeat them many times. They are acting like a stabilizing "smoother" *(Figure 2 – Landmark 4)*.

f) Finish this treatment by a harmonization of the third chakra using the Umbrella Method *(Landmark 5)*.

Note: This treatment is practiced indifferently on the back or the front of the body.

12) "Psychological" readjustment of the subtle bodies

It happens that people are having misaligned subtle bodies to their physical body for a long period of time. This pathology is often created by important emotional and affective shocks experienced as well as the rejection of a specific situation and/or a flight facing some aspects of daily reality.

a) This treatment is preferably practiced in supine position. Bring the second and third chakras in resonance using The Solar Circulation. Do the same with the fifth and the sixth chakras, and then the first chakra, which will happen at a distance for obvious reasons, and the coronal (seventh chakra). Do worry about the polarity of your hands (Landmark 1, 2 and 3).

b) With The Umbrella Method, reharmonize the cardiac chakra.

   To reharmonize, keep your hand flat on this chakra. With closed eyes, visualize, for a long time, concentric circles spreading slowly from a point on a liquid surface (Landmark 4 & 5).

c) Resume then, phase by phase, the whole treatment of the mechanical realignment.

13) Coccygeal memories

The tail bone is certainly one of the areas of the body that is most difficult to treat, not only because of its anatomical location but also because of what it "contains" on the vibrational plan. It is indeed a region where many memories are concentrated, of which implications can be impulsive, emotional, affective and spiritual.

Behind and under it, the therapist is directly in contact with the kundalini force, a fearsome reservoir of energy coiled up on itself.

Touching the coccyx is far from insignificant. The therapist will only intervene in this area with infinite precautions and with the client's agreement.

The intervention is only justified when the client feels blocked in his inner advance, facing his fears, his stubborn symptoms, difficultly analyzed then, and often facing annoying reactive behaviors to live for himself.

When the person to heal had the sensation of stagnation in his own life, the Essenian and Egyptian therapists treated the coccygeal area to arouse illuminating visions or liberating dreams.

Absolutely avoid this treatment on people who refuse a challenge to their way of life.

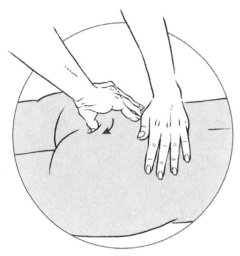

Figure 1

a) With full respect, you place your thumb of your active hand on the base of the tail bone of your client. Once you feel the base well, move your thumb slightly towards his left, where you perceive a slight indentation. Massage very gently this point using small clockwise movements.

Meanwhile, the other fingers of your active hand support the sacrum. As for your supportive hand, you place it horizontally on the lumbar region *(Figure 1)*.

Do the same thing on the right side of the coccyx and finally on its central extremity.

The pressure of your thumb on these three points must be moderate and consider the potential pain experienced by your client.

b) From the exacting base of the coccyx, the thumb of your active hand will move up slowly towards the sacrum by maintaining its pressure, while your supportive hand will position vertically to move up along the dorsal axis with the same rhythm *(Figure 2)*.

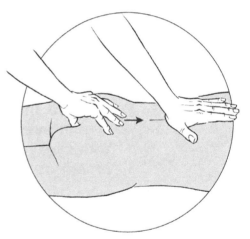

Figure 2

c) Arrived at the sacrum, your active hand will land flat on it. Then move it up very gently on the dorsal axis just below your supportive hand, which, then will carry it slowly in its movement to the cardiac chakra *(Figure 3)*.

d) You complete this treatment by putting in resonance according to the usual method of The Solar Circulation, the second and fourth chakras.

Suggested oils (always dilute): "Chakra 7", "Chakra 1", "Revealing", Spruce Hemlock Essential Oil, Spike Essential Oil, and Myrrh of Essential Oil.

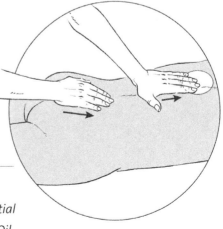

Figure 3

**Dare dreaming the Universe
That dwells secretly within you,
Dare project It outside of you,
To make it into a world,
Because, in truth, It is the quality
of your eyes that creates,
Your eyes have hands in the
consciousness of the Eternal.**[24]

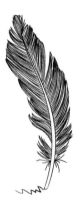

NINTH PART

Techniques Used in Specific Treatments

A ncient therapists conceived the techniques used in specific treatments to treat well defined disorders that affect organs and systems. Numerous pathologies identified and analyzed by modern medicine were not known as such thousands of years ago. For example, we didn't talk about diabetes, hypertension or thyroid problems. However, this does not mean the symptoms related to these conditions were unknown and were not the subject of research in studies of the subtle functioning of the human being.

The following pages introduce a number of protocols carried out by therapists according to the energetic origin of the most common disorders they encountered, which modern medicine has given particular names.

The list of therapies is not exhaustive—it is likely to develop over the years with the discoveries made in the Akashic records.

1) COLOPATHY AND INTESTINAL DYSFUNCTION

This treatment, which addresses chronic problems in particular, is intended to heal general intestinal disorders without distinguishing the nature of the disorders. It involves a technique of regulation of the total function of the colon. Don't assume it simply masks a disorder—it touches on what the Ancient Ones called "the intestinal intelligence of the being" by trying to restore the balance of the energetic exchanges that play a part in the mechanism of excretion.

The notion of "intelligence of the organism" was constantly present by the Essenians and Egyptians. The concept refers to the functioning of the body capable of escaping our mental analysis, whatever its level of refinement.

a) Place your client in a supine position. After creating an Operative Field on the person's abdomen, make two big etheric incisions. These incisions must follow the path of the great nadis that intersect as shoulder straps by drawing an X where the center is located, more or less at the navel, with the extremities at the last floating ribs and the iliac crests* *(Landmark 1).*

b) Once you have created these two big etheric openings according to the method described previously,** use your active hand to delicately open the etheric abdomen of your client by lifting the four parts you have marked using small movements similar to those you would use when peeling an orange. You must feel and grab the etheric matter between your fingers *(Landmark 2).*

c) The etheric abdomen of your client is then fully "open." Using the Method of Three Fingers Unified, consciously brush the whole opening with Light. To do this, use the tips of your fingers to draw circles or arcs from right to left and left to right. Spend more time on the superior half of the opening *(Landmark 3).*

d) Internalize and remove your astral hand from your physical hand to let it gently penetrate the entire mass of the colon. Infuse it with Light and love *(Landmark 4).*

e) Carefully fold back the four parts of the big etheric opening you created and, once closed, smooth the lips of the wound *(Landmark 5).*

* See Map of Nadis p. 29.
** See p. 69.

f) Reharmonize the third and fifth chakras, and then bring resonance between them using Solar Circulation *(Landmarks 6, 7 and 8)*.

g) Take the soles of your client's feet between your hands and transmit to the person all the force of anchoring possible *(Landmark 9)*.

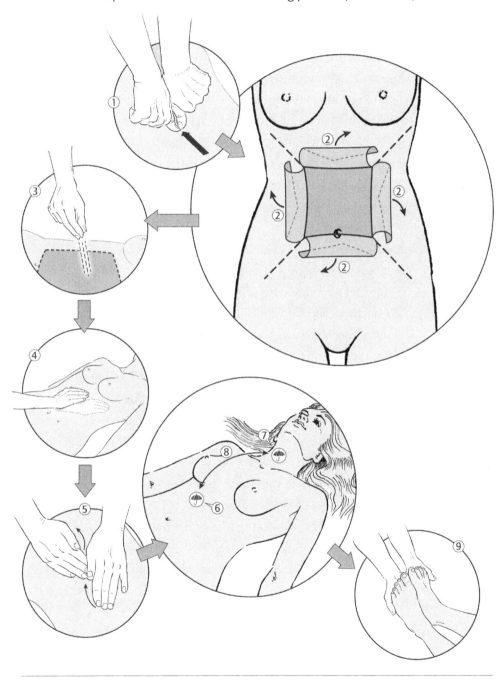

Suggested oils (always dilute): "Emotional Balance", "Letting Go", "Chakra 1", Spruce Hemlock Essential oil and Lavandula officinalis Essential Oil

2) INTESTINAL DISORDERS

This treatment is designed specifically for temporary intestinal problems such as irritation, diarrhea, colitis and so forth.

a) Start by creating an Operative Field in the traditional manner on the entire abdomen *(Figure 1, Landmark 1)*.

b) Make an Etheric Incision in the abdomen by following the diagonals that cross it by forming straps. Then, grab the etheric matter and lift each triangle created toward the outside to generate a big, subtle opening over the entire intestinal mass, like in the colopathy treatment *(Landmark 2)*.

c) After internalizing, slide your disembodied active astral hand into the opening you have made. If possible, slide in the other hand in the same way *(Landmark 3)*.

Two phases follow:
  - Internally visualize a sun in the center of your cardiac chakra, and feel how it radiates until it engulfs you and your client. Ask for healing before letting it gently shrink its solar radiance into your cardiac chakra.
  - Center yourself on the laryngeal chakra. Perceive it radiating a distinct blue wave that is being transmitted to your arm(s) and hand(s). Feel this blue wave expand throughout your client's abdomen and renew your call for healing *(Landmark 3)*.

d) Remove your subtle hand or hands from your client's abdomen. Close and smooth the etheric wound you created *(Landmark 4)*.

e) Reharmonize the third chakra in the traditional way *(Figure 2, Landmark 5)*.

f) Move to your client's feet and take the person's soles in your hands. Infuse them with the energy of healing *(Landmark 6)*.

g) Create resonance using Solar Circulation in the fourth and fifth chakras *(Landmark 7)*.

Suggested oils (always dilute): "Emotional Balance", "Letting Go", "Chakra 1", Basil Essential Oil, Spruce Hemlock Essential Oil and Lavandula officinalis Essential Oil

---

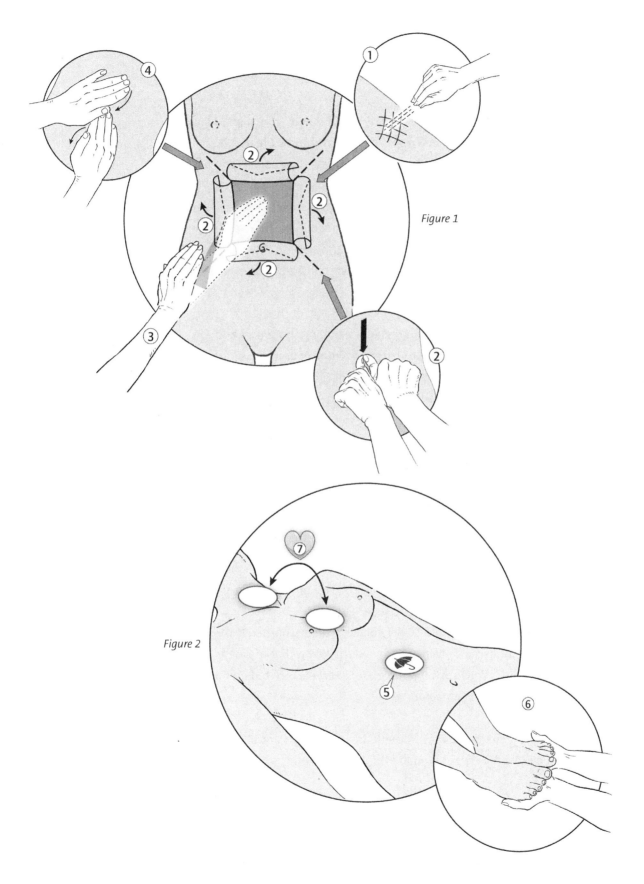

Figure 1

Figure 2

3) RECURRING THROAT PROBLEMS

This treatment aims to reinforce the immune defenses and work locally with the goal of disinfection.

a) Make an Etheric Incision in each side of the throat, from a point located 1.18 inches (3 centimeters) from the base of the ear. Create two openings from this point to the cartilage of the glottis *(Adam's apple; Landmark 1)*.

b) Using the traditional Method of Three Fingers Unified, infuse the energy of healing by making small movements from top to bottom and bottom to top. Then, close the two etheric wounds and smooth them *(Landmark 2)*.
   Practice this treatment on both sides of the throat even if only one side is affected.

c) Create an Operative Field* on the area including the spleen and the pancreas. Make a big Etheric Incision. After profound internalization, practice the method of disembodiment of the astral hand (active) by entering the opening you just created. Infuse the area with the energy of healing *(Landmarks 3 and 4)*.

d) While your astral arm remains in contact with the subtle spleen and pancreas, place your supportive hand on the etheric part of your client's laryngeal chakra and slowly allow it to touch the skin *(Landmark 5)*.

e) Circulate the energy of healing from your heart to your active hand and, afterward, to your client's throat, where your supportive hand remains. Send back this energy to your heart. The wave of healing must circulate freely in loop as long as you feel it necessary.
   You will notice that this circulation can be counterclockwise and that it is not necessarily like the Solar Circulation that moves according to which hand is active or supportive. Our example is based on the right hand being active *(Landmark 6)*.

f) Slowly remove your hands from the treated areas. Carefully close and smooth the big etheric wound over the spleen and pancreas *(Landmark 7)*.

g) Harmonize the throat chakra using The Method of the Umbrella, and bring this chakra in resonance with the sixth using Solar Circulation *(Landmarks 8 and 9)*.

* See p. 68.

Ideally, you should initiate a discussion with your client to determine the mental or emotional causes of the throat problem (thought forms, mental crystallizations, fear, anger, etc.). Using the Archetypes is desirable.**

Note: This treatment, which can be used for repetitive anginas, for example, can also be efficient for simple chronic hoarseness.

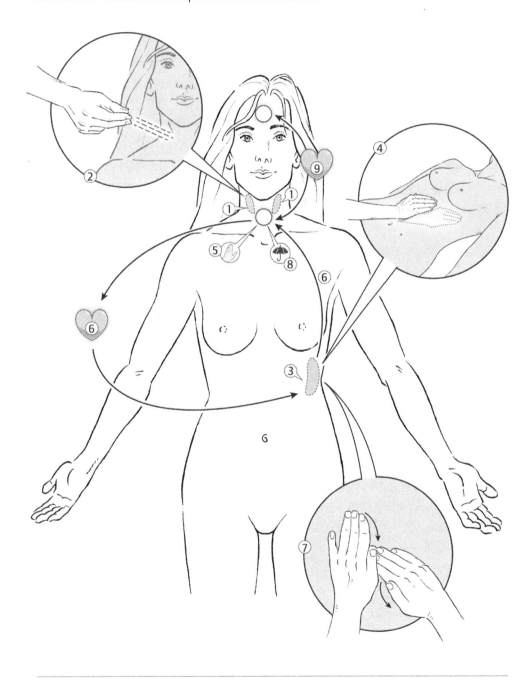

Suggested oils (always dilute): "Expression", "Joy", Spruce Hemlock Essential Oil, rose of Damascus Essential Oil and Lavandula officinalis Essential Oil

** See p. 170.

4) THERAPY RELATED TO THE LARYNGEAL CHAKRA

We regularly encounter people who suffer from energetic blockages at the level of the throat. The main source of their suffering often comes from failure to express their feelings. The therapy here is exclusively Essenian. The Essenians focused on developing this therapy because they understood the art of oral expression. The especially favored "the voice of milk" because of its liberating and balancing effect.

This treatment is particularly powerful. It is also complicated, and it requires good fluidity in its mastery. Moreover, it is remarkable because of the softness it involves—a client crying after treatment is not unusual.

With your client in a supine position, stand on the person's right side. For this treatment, you do not have to consider your active and supportive hands. Only the notion of right and left is important.

Before starting the actual treatment, apply a conifer oil—ideally hemlock oil—to the secondary chakra on the client's right wrist, to the one on the right shoulder and, finally, to the one on the throat.

a) With your left hand, hold your client's right arm. Meanwhile, delicately massage the secondary chakra of the person's wrist with the flat of your fingers using a clockwise motion. This effleurage of the area of the pulse can trigger emotion by itself *(Figure 1)*.

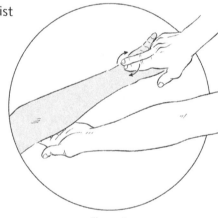

Figure 1

b) While your left hand remains under your client's right arm, position the fingers of your right hand at your client's right fingertips; by doing so, infuse all the wave of Light you can. This wave will move up along your client's arm. Let it expand, and then gently slide your flat hand along the person's forearm until your fingertips reach the secondary chakra of the elbow. Pause here, with your hand still flat. You are about to reverse the normal flow of the forearm, which tends to cause the energy to unload *(Figure 2)*.

c) Slide your left hand under your client's right shoulder. With one or two fingers of your right hand, massage the secondary chakra of your client's right shoulder using small clockwise movements *(Figure 3)*.

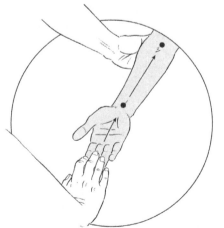

Figure 2

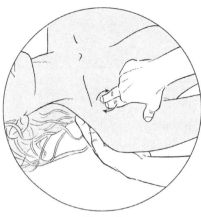

Figure 3

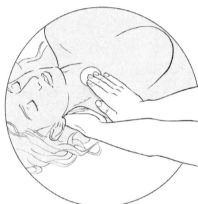

Figure 4

d) Slide your left hand under your client's neck. Simultaneously place your right hand horizontally so that it follows the energetic circuit that unifies the secondary chakra of the shoulder with the laryngeal chakra (fifth chakra). Infuse the wave of healing for a few moments before employing Solar Circulation *(Figure 4)*.

e) With your left hand still under your client's neck, place the United Three Fingers of your right hand in the client's area of energetic contact above the laryngeal chakra. Then, perform an unscrewing movement on the pistil of the chakra with the help of your fingertips, moving counterclockwise. In addition to these movements, make slow clockwise movements with your hand around the global area of the chakra. Maintaining two opposite movements at the same time requires skill. However, learn to master this technique because it is crucial. We will call it the Method of the Screwdriver *(Figures 5 and 5 bis)*.

f) Harmonize the laryngeal chakra using The Method of the Umbrella *(Figure 6, Landmark 1)*.

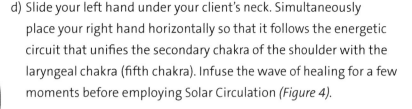

g) On the right and left sides of the client's body, gently massage in a clockwise direction the three points indicated on the schema* *(Figure 6, Landmarks 2, 3 and 4)*.

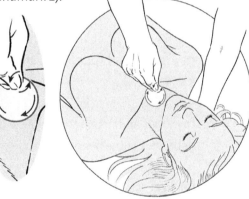

Figure 5

h) Harmonize the third chakra by means of The Method of the Umbrella *(Figure 6, Landmark 5)*.

i) You traditionally finish this treatment by placing your hands in the shape of a T on the area of the laryngeal chakra.**

Suggested oils (always dilute): "Expression", "Emotional Balance", Spruce Hemlock Essential Oil and Petit grain Essential Oil

* See Map of the Nadis on p. 29.
** See p. 87, Figure 2.

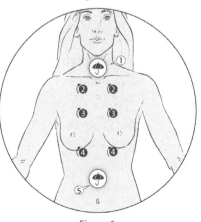

Figure 6

5) THE REGULATION OF THE THYROID

This treatment is for both hypo- and hyperthyroidism. Like all Essene–Egyptian treatments, it is not destined to "fight" the problem but to reestablish a balance in a way we cannot comprehend.

- *Hypothyroidism* often results from a slowing of the general metabolism, fatigue, chilliness, memory disorders and a tendency to constipation.
- *Hyperthyroidism* is mainly manifested by weight loss, diarrhea, sleeping disorders, mood disorders and heat intolerance.

To practice this treatment effectively, the therapist must know the correct location of the thyroid, what it looks like with its two lobes, and its subtle relationship with the laryngeal chakra, Vishuddha and the mental body.

a) You start by harmonizing the cardiac chakra using The Method of the Umbrella *(Figure 1, Landmark 1)*.

b) Place the united emissive three fingers of your active hand on the space of radiance above the forehead chakra (sixth chakra) and practice The Method of the Dropper to offer it to this chakra.

c) Do the same, using the same method (The Dropper), at the level of the right lobe of your client's thyroid, and then on the left lobe, too *(Landmark 3)*.

d) Lay your hand flat on the laryngeal chakra and call the green light to be deposited at the heart of this chakra with your exhalation *(Landmark 4)*.

e) With the United Three Fingers of your hand, practice the Method of the Screwdriver on each lobe of the thyroid *(Figure 2, Landmark 5)*.

f) Harmonize the laryngeal chakra in the traditional way, and then introduce resonance with the seventh chakra according to The Solar Circulation technique *(Landmarks 6 and 7)*.

Suggested oils (always dilute): "Expression" and Rose of Damascus Essential Oil and Spruce Hemlock Essential Oil

---

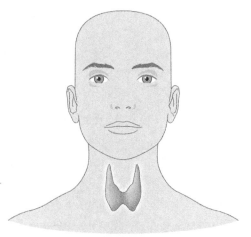

LOCATION OF THE THYROID
with its two lobes

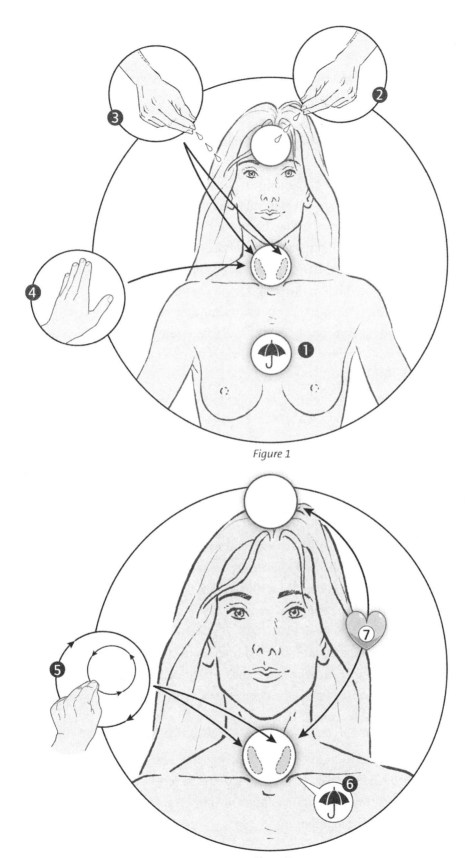

Figure 1

Figure 2

6) DIABETES

Diabetes has two essential causes:

- Partial or total incapacity of the pancreas to synthetize insulin
- Inability of the cells to deliver insulin for glucose absorption

Because it is not well absorbed by the cells, glucose can concentrate in the blood and lead to hyperglycemia, or an increase in the glucose concentration in the blood.

In addition, there are two types of diabetes:

- *Type 1 diabetes*, previously known as juvenile diabetes, occurs in about 10% of cases. This condition is characterized by the pancreas producing too little, or no, insulin, possibly due to a virus, but mostly due to emotional schema.
- *Type 2 diabetes* occurs in about 90% of cases. This condition appears when the body shows insulin resistance; that is, the body doesn't use insulin properly and it cannot keep up with the demand for insulin required to regulate blood glucose levels.

We must understand that insulin regulates the glycemic rate in the blood. Even if diabetes had not been identified thousands of years ago, people still experienced its symptoms and dangers.

The following treatment essentially helps for type 1 diabetes. However, we can practice it on clients with type 2 diabetes, especially if it is rooted in the emotions.

a) Start by harmonizing your client's third chakra using The Method of the Umbrella *(Figure 1, Landmark 1)*.

b) Practice the antistress* movement at least three consecutive times. The movement involves using the thumb of your active hand to create a circular arc between the subchakra of the last left floating rib and the point located above the left breast *(Landmark 2)*.

c) You can now choose to practice either the etheric extraction of the pancreas** or its penetration using an extension of the astral hand. In both cases, it is essential to feel the energetic mass of the organ in your hand *(Figure 2, Landmark 4)*.

d) The next step is a crucial phase that can be broken into two parts:
   1) Once you have established contact with the pancreas, practice on it the Method of Solar Circulation on it by reversing its sense. Infuse a dynamic momentum.

* See p. 100.
** See p. 71.

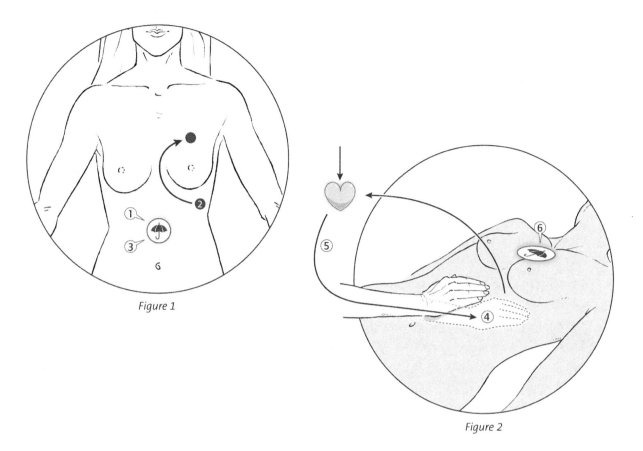

Figure 1

Figure 2

2) As soon as this first loop is accomplished, practice again the same circular movement but with an interior calming breath (Landmark 5).

Repeat the two phases, 1) then 2), as many times as you feel necessary. The pancreas will thus receive, alternately, a tonic influx and a softening breath. It is crucial to understand and execute the double intention of the reversed Solar Circulation. This is the heart of this practice.

e) Finally, finish your treatment by applying The Method of the Umbrella to the heart chakra (Landmark 6).

Cover your client with a blanket and allow time for recovery, as this treatment may leave the person "shaken".

Suggested oils (always dilute): "Emotional Balance", "Serenity", Rose of Damascus Essential Oil, Lavandula officinalis Essential Oil, chamomile Essential Oil and Petit grain Essential Oil.

7) HIGH BLOOD PRESSURE

Hypertension is defined as the consequence of too much tension of the blood on the arterial walls. It is not a disease in a strict sense but rather an important risk factor that could lead to the deterioration of one's health.

Indeed, it can cause cardiac insufficiency (fatigue of the muscle), infarctions, cerebrovascular strokes, arteriosclerosis (fragility of arteries), renal failure and retinal lesions due to the fragility of blood vessels. Its main causes include old age, stress, genetic factors, a sedentary lifestyle, smoking, alcoholism, obesity and ingesting too much salt.

The Essenians and Egyptians, who knew the symptoms, although to a lesser extent than we do, tackled the problem in the following manner:

a) Start by placing your active hand on the secondary chakra of the right shoulder of your client and your supportive hand on the last right floating rib. Create resonance between these two points using solar circulation *(Figure 1, Landmark 1)*.

b) Do the same on the left side of the body *(Landmark 2)*.

c) Now, place your supportive hand on the point of the right iliac crest and your active hand on the point of the last left floating rib. You thus create a diagonal. Then, employ Solar Circulation *(Landmark 3)*.

d) Repeat, this time placing your supportive hand on the left iliac crest and your active hand on the last right floating rib. This creates a second energetic diagonal on the abdomen *(Landmark 4)*.

e) Now, create resonance. Always use the same method: placing the supportive hand on the point of the right iliac crest and the active hand on the right shoulder. Likewise, bring resonance to the same points on the left side of the client's body *(Landmarks 5 and 6)*.

f) Create the same resonance by placing your supportive hand on the sole of the right foot and your active hand on the second chakra. Repeat it on the left side *(Landmarks 7 and 8)*.

g) Bring a last resonance to the third and fourth chakras, with your active hand on the fourth chakra, the one of the heart *(Landmark 9)*.

Suggested oils (always dilute): "Quietude", "Heart", Rose of Damascus Essential oil and Lavandula officinalis Essential Oil.

h) Finally, place your supportive hand under your client's neck and, simultaneously with The Method of the Umbrella, harmonize the cardiac chakra with your active hand *(Figure 2, Landmark 10)*.

Note: To avoid moving too often around your client, you can complete steps e) and f) after one another on one side before moving to the other side. It will thus be easier to consider the polarity of each hand because you should never cross your hands in this or any other treatment.

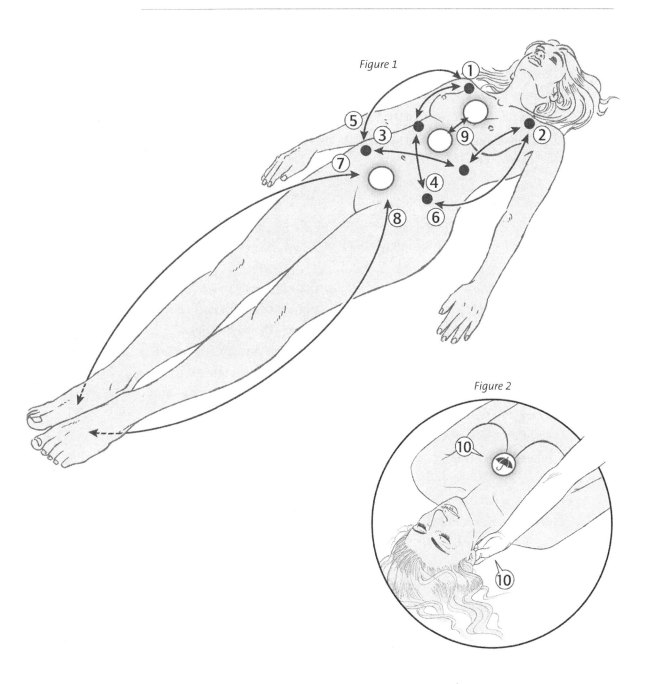

Figure 1

Figure 2

8) CHRONIC RENAL INSUFFICIENCY

Chronic renal insufficiency is an important progressive and definitive decrease of blood filtration by the kidneys. This leads to the retention of waste as, for example, urea. This insufficiency is induced by pathologies such as diabetes and hypertension that progressively destroy the different renal structures. The last phase requires dialysis or receiving a transplant.

a) Start by creating an energetic resonance on the second and fifth chakras of your client. You can lay your active hand on either *(Figure 1, Landmark 1)*.

b) Position yourself at the midpoint of the client's calves, and massage the secondary chakras and the two iliac crests slowly but firmly with your thumbs, simultaneously and clockwise. Without releasing the pressure, bring your thumbs down to the soles of the feet by following the path of the major nadis of the legs (groin, mid-thigh, knee, calf and heel) *(Landmarks 2 and 3)*.

c) Take your client's right foot in your active hand and lay your supportive hand on the second chakra. Infuse the wave of healing from the feet to the chakra, and do the same from the left foot *(Landmarks 4 and 5)*.

d) On the anterior side but slightly to the right side of the client's abdomen, and after applying an Operative Field, create an Etheric Incision, and then open a wound in the subtle tissues according the method described previously. Internalize yourself to detach your astral hand, and then slide your astral hand into the opening you created, through the intestinal mass, to wrap the right kidney. Diffuse the most beautiful wave of love as long as it seems necessary. Gently remove your subtle hand and then close the etheric wound carefully. Treat the left kidney the same way *(Figure 2, Landmark 6)*.

e) Place your hands on the lateral and anterior sides of each kidney and bring them, one after another, into resonance with the second chakra by Solar Circulation *(Landmark 7)*.

f) Ideally, finish with an Archetypal treatment according to the method described at the end of this book. Determine which treatment to use at the beginning of the session during a discussion with your client.

Suggested oils (always dilute): "Revelation", "Kidneys", "Chakra 6", Lavandula officinalis Essential Oil, Spikenard Essential Oil and Frankincense Essential Oil.

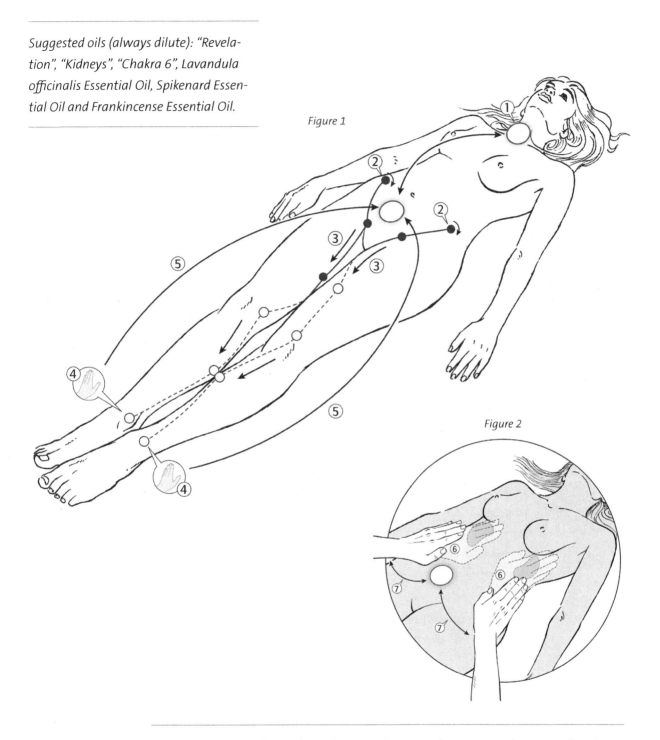

Figure 1

Figure 2

Note: The clients suffering from this pathology are often naïve and emotional and have difficulty using discernment. Therefore, we could refer to line 13 of the Table of the Archetypes, but in exceptional cases, we will trace the Hebraic M on the physical body at the sixth chakra and at the parallel lines four times in the emotional aura of the same chakra.

9) Sleep apnea

a) Start by making a full-length ethereal incision on the client's diaphragm to create a subtle opening according the method learned *(Figure 1, Landmark 1).*

b) Detach your astral active hand and introduce it gently into the right part of the client's diaphragm. Do the same on the left side. With compassion, infuse Light and relaxation *(Landmarks 2 and 3).*

c) After closing the Etheric Incision of the diaphragm, create another one vertically from the epigastrium to the navel. Slide you astral active hand in vertically with the same loving attitude and while considering the shaped dome of the diaphragm. Close the etheric wound and smooth it *(Figure 2, Landmarks 4 and 5).*

d) Harmonize the third and fifth chakras using The Method of the Umbrella and create resonance using Solar Circulation.

e) With the unified three fingers of your active hand, use The Wave of Healing to infuse the points located on each side of the client's nostrils, slightly toward their bottom ends *(Figure 3, Landmarks 9 and 10).*

f) Do the same at the level of the point located in the center of the base of the nose *(Landmark 11).*

g) Create resonance using Solar Circulation on the nadis crossing like two suspenders on the rib cage *(Landmarks 12 and 13).*

h) End your treatment by performing a traditional harmonization of the cardiac chakra of your client *(Landmark 14).*

Suggested oils (always dilute): "Letting Go", Lavandula officinalis Essential Oil, Rose of Damascus Essential Oil, Spruce Hemlock Essential Oil and Myrrh Essential Oil.

When the eyes are the extension of the soul, they collect the honey that wherein they touch down.[28]

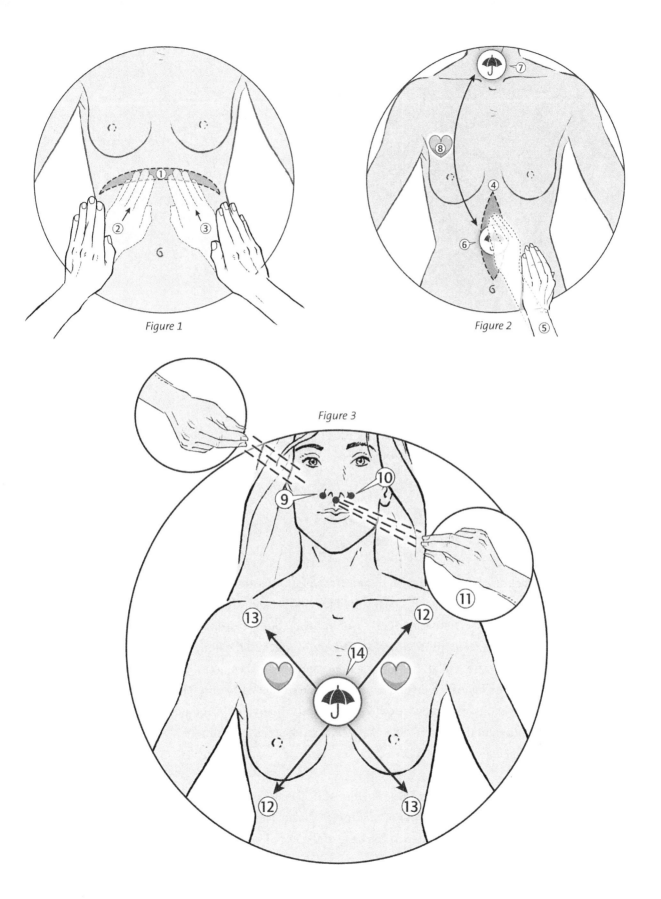

Figure 1

Figure 2

Figure 3

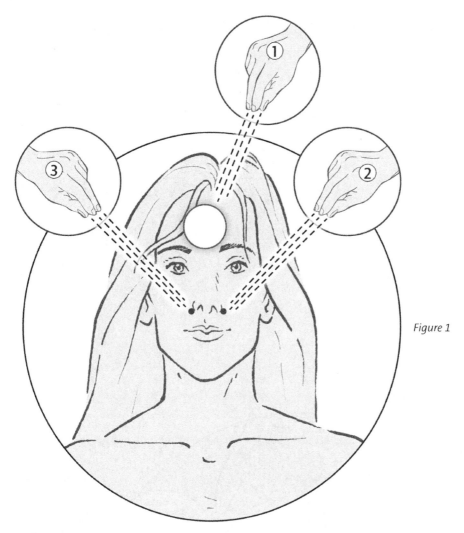

Figure 1

10) ASTHMA

There are three types of asthma: chronic asthma, stress-induced asthma and allergy-related asthma. This treatment is best suited for chronic and stress-related asthma. In both cases, we can treat the condition at intervals, but it is desirable to apply it regularly over several months to have a substantial effect on the body.

Regarding asthma from allergies, the Essenians and Egyptians practically ignored it because of the radical difference in their lifestyle compared to ours. They experienced little exposure to substances or foods that cause allergies. With this condition, it is best to treat the cause of the allergy. Nevertheless, the treatment described here could be a significant aid.

    a) With the help of the United Three Fingers, start by infusing the luminous wave of healing into the center of the frontal chakra. Next, infuse it precisely at each point located at the base of the nostrils *(Figure 1, Landmarks 1, 2 and 3).*

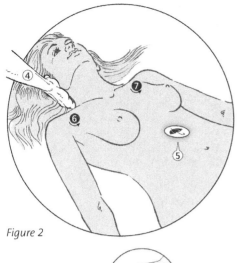

Figure 2

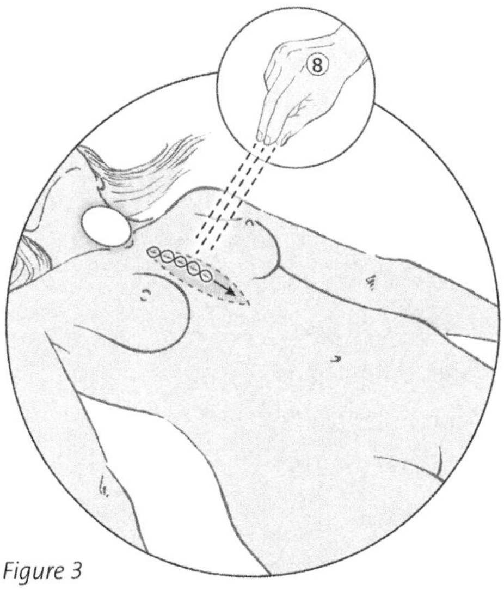

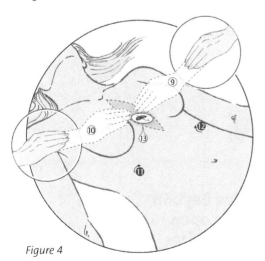

Figure 3

b) Place your supportive hand under your client's neck and, simultaneously, practice the reharmonization of the third chakra using the traditional Method of the Umbrella *(Figure 2, Landmarks 4 and 5).*

c) Massage the secondary chakras of the shoulders in a counterclockwise direction *(Landmarks 6 and 7).*

d) Make an Etheric Incision from the laryngeal chakra to the epigastrium and again use your United Three Fingers to infuse a luminous beam in the subtle wound. With the help of the Wave of Healing, trace a series of small lemniscates, or infinity symbols, very slowly from top to bottom. Repeat these movements as many times as you feel necessary.

e) With the greatest gentleness and internalization, slide your active hand into the astral extension and then into the opening. This will infuse the Wave of Healing at the top of the client's bronchi, first the right and then the left. Don't forget to close and smooth the etheric wound afterward *(Figure 4, Landmarks 9 and 10).*

f) Massage clockwise the subchakra of each floating rib *(Landmarks 11 and 12).*

g) Reharmonize the cardiac chakra *(Landmark 13).*

h) Ideally, you should consider working with the Archetypes, as indicated at the end of this book. We suggest, for most cases, you refer to line 5 of the Table of the Archetypes. On the client's body at the fifth chakra, trace the Hebraic symbol that corresponds to the letter E three times; then, in the etheric of the fifth chakra, trace a triangle five times. At line 6, trace the Hebraic "Vau" on the sixth chakra three times, and finally, in the etheric of the sixth chakra, trace parallel lines six times.

Figure 4

Suggested oils (always dilute): "Lucidity", "Chakra 6", "Expression", Spruce hemlock Essential Oil and Rose of Damascus Essential Oil

11) ARTICULAR RHEUMATISM

Of course, this treatment can be applied to any joint affected by rheumatism, but we have chosen to use a knee joint as example.

a) Start the treatment by balancing the second chakra according to the Umbrella Method *(Figure 1, Landmark 1)*.

b) Set up an Operative Field on the affected area *(Landmark 2)*.

c) Internalize yourself deeply and let your active astral hand penetrate the painful joint (without any Etheric Incision). As soon as your hand subtly penetrates this joint, infuse a luminous wave that you internally color white, then green, then mauve, then again white, green, mauve, and so forth. Respect the order of these colors, and feel each of their phases. Their cycles must be slow and clearly perceived from within. Carefully remove your astral hand *(Landmark 3)*.

d) Simultaneously place your supportive hand flat on the treatment area and your active hand on the second chakra. Internally seek the etheric snags accumulated in the affective area using your supportive hand, bring them up through your arm, transit them to your cardiac chakra, and bring them down to the second chakra via your active arm in the form of a white. This will complete the energetic recycling of the snags using your cardiac chakra. Close the loop by sending a Wave of Healing through the nadis of the leg to the affected area, still with your supportive hand. Repeat this loop fluidly as long you feel is necessary. In the case of our example, its movement is the reverse of Solar Circulation *(Figure 2, Landmarks 4 and 5)*.

Suggested oils (always dilute): "Revealing", "Letting Go" and Spruce Hemlock.

Each soul contains a mystery that we can't perceive beyond a certain point. We must accept that doors partially open by themselves in a timely manner, by laughing at our desires and at our impatience. There is what we want and what we need, and only an abandonment of our warrior resistances allows us to see and accept the nuance between them.[29]

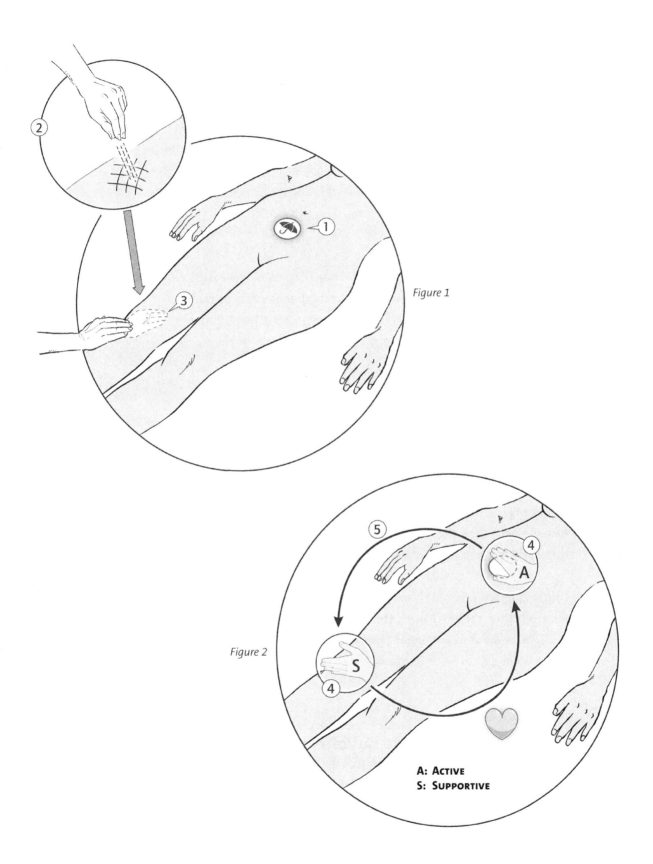

Figure 1

Figure 2

A: Active
S: Supportive

12) Strains, sprains and elongations

a) First of all, it is correct to gently massage all the energy points located above and below the wounded area in a counterclockwise direction. For our example, we have chosen the elbow joint *(Figure 1, Landmark 1).*

b) Depending on the extent of the affected area, practice three or four etheric incisions above the wounded area to access a large number of micronadis. Once you have created the etheric opening, infuse the Wave of Healing into it and then close it carefully before going to the next opening *(Landmarks 2 and 3).*

c) Place your active hand flat on the global zone that has been incised, fingers directed toward the affected joint. Simultaneously slide your supportive hand under it perpendicularly to your active hand. In this example, the therapist is positioned toward the head of the client *(Figure 2, Landmark 4).*

d) While maintaining this position, internalize yourself, specially calling the Light within you, and begin to set in motion Solar Circulation starting from your heart. The wave will be transmitted to your supportive hand, which will move it to your active hand through the wounded area and so on.

    At each of your slow inhalations, visualize a clear green light; meanwhile, at each of your exhalations, cultivate the sensation of firmly extracting the dark green waste. Always breathe in and out through the nose *(Landmark 5).*

e) Form a cone with your unified hands above the wounded joint for a few moments then perform etheric smoothing of the entire treated area.

    Repeat this treatment as often possible because it aims to accelerate the recovery of the damaged tissues.

The pure soul doesn't calculate but offers without counting: the pure soul doesn't know the sinuosity, but offers the transparency; the soul who is pure never expects the time to make prayers, it is always the prayer offered by the hands; it is always the hands which serve and the ones who receive the Light.[30]

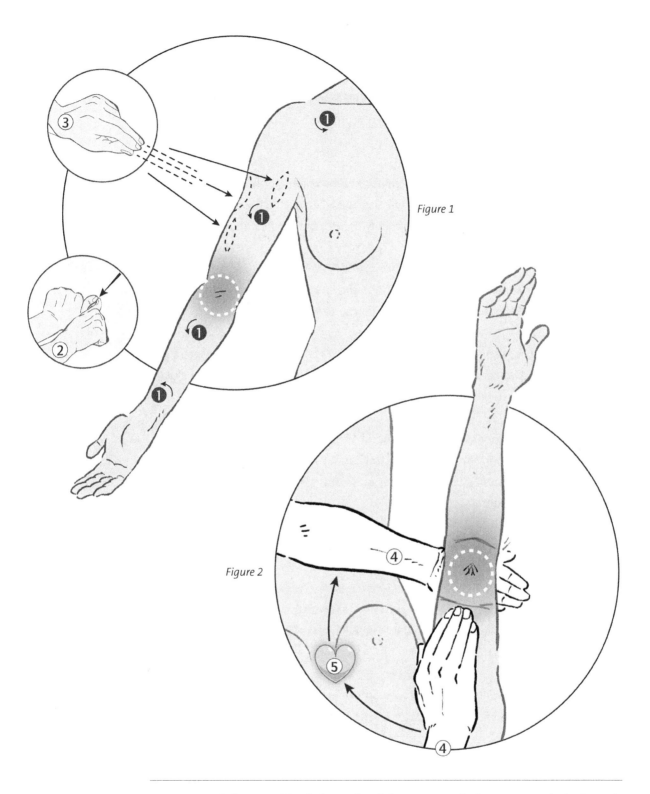

Figure 1

Figure 2

Suggested oils (always dilute): "Revealing", "Repairing Balm", Spruce Hemlock of Essential Oil and Lavandula officinalis Essential Oil.

13) Fibromyalgia

Fibromyalgia is characterized by a chronic muscular pain accompanied by chronic fatigue. Although most sufferers are women, an increasing number of men are reporting suffering from this condition. This treatment from the Essenians and the Egyptians, who had analyzed the symptoms, can be used to reinforce a weakened system.

a) First, position yourself at the client's head and gently take the person's neck in the palms of your hands. Use Solar Circulation to invoke a luminous wave that benefits mainly the cerebellum *(Figure 1, Landmark 1)*.

b) With a tonifying oil, trace small lemniscates on the front face of the channels of Ida and Pingala between the laryngeal chakra and the cardiac chakra. Repeat this many times *(Figure 2, Landmarks 2 and 3)*.

c) Place your supportive hand on the laryngeal chakra and, simultaneously, on the cardiac chakra. Bring these two centers in resonance through Solar Circulation while visualizing a green light *(Landmark 4)*.

d) Create an Etheric Incision at the level of the spleen before using the method of detachment of the astral hand. Your subtle hand must make energetic contact with the etheric mass of the spleen. Ideally, it infuses an orange light.

e) Reharmonize the second and fifth chakras using The Umbrella Method *(Landmarks 6 and 7)*.
   Only when possible, and when it is easy to understand why, place your supportive hand flat on the laryngeal chakra while you infuse a luminous wave with The Unified Three Fingers of your active hand at the level of the perineum.

Suggested oils (always dilute): "Vitality", Joy, Spruce Hemlock Essential Oil, Neroli Essential Oil, and Rose of Damascus Essential Oil

---

If the Divine is our origin, It is also our common resultant. We are nourishing It.[26]

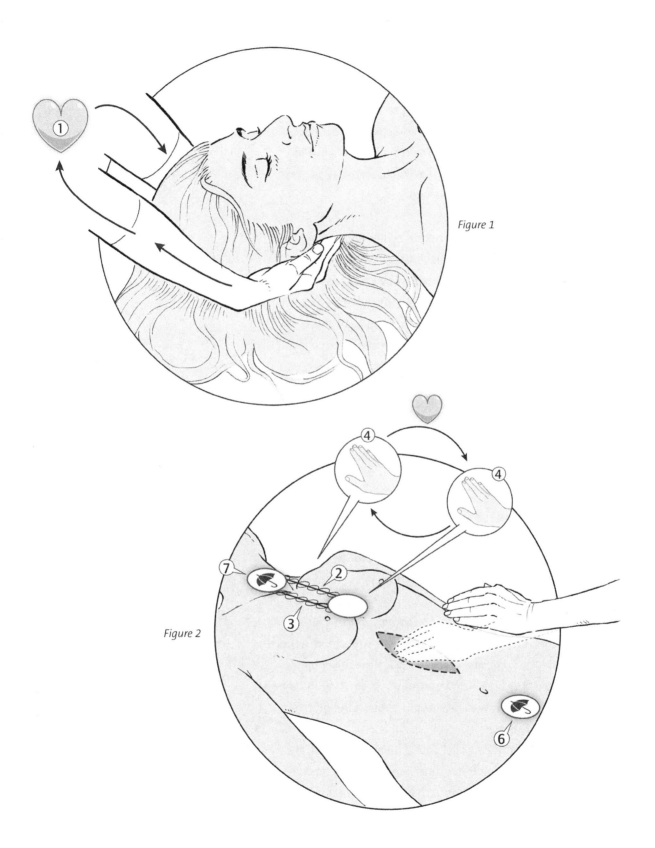

Figure 1

Figure 2

14) Sleeping disorders

a) Start by positioning yourself at the client's head and laying your forehead on the person to "scan" his or her body from top to bottom according to the method described in this book.* Don't practice this method in a neutral manner as we should usually do, but focus your awareness on the concept of insomnia. Note the major point where you have the sensation of "being blocked" *(Landmark 1)*.

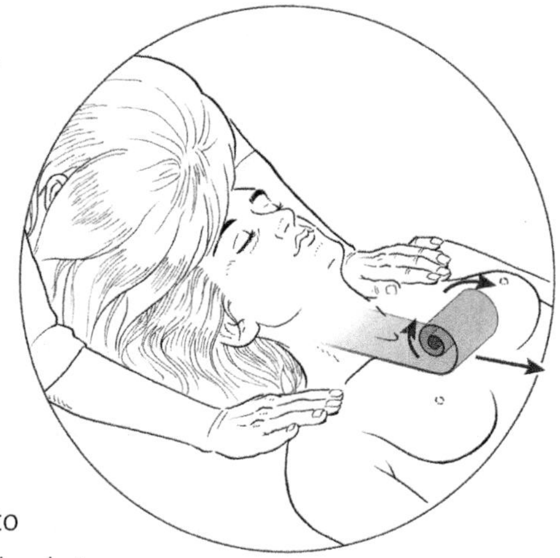

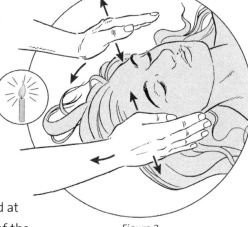

Figure 1

b) Stay at the head of your client but straighten up. Place each of your hands at the level of the client's temples to create slight physical contact. Move away from them slowly to enter the etheric temporal area. By doing this, create small lateral movements back and forth and front to back as if to palpate the ether. Your intention must be to collect, and unstick the etheric snags that are inevitably stagnant in cases of repeated insomnia. Carry on until you obtain a sensation of fluidity. Once finished, it is imperative that you clean your hands by passing them over the flame of a candle *(Figure 2)*.

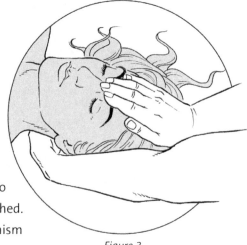

Figure 2

c) Slide your supportive hand under the client's neck and place your active hand on the person's forehead at the same time, fingers oriented toward the bridge of the nose. Ask for Light and help *(Figure 3)*.

d) Leave the client's head and position yourself on one of the person's sides. Slide your supportive hand under the neck and gradually place the other hand on the area identified by scanning. If you weren't able to identify any area, place your active hand on the area of the liver.

    In both cases, let your active hand penetrate astrally (without Etheric Incision) the concerned area to smooth it internally once the subtle contact is established. Remove your astral hand gently from the client's organism *(Figure 4, Landmark 1)*.

Figure 3

* See p. 125.

e) Clean the throat chakra deeply using the Technique of the Screwdriver studied previously,* then reharmonize it with The Method of the Umbrella (*Figure 4, Landmarks 2 and 3*).

f) Smooth the entire subtle body, first firmly and then gently, several times from top to bottom. Finish with a traditional harmonization of the cardiac chakra (*Figure 5, Landmarks 4 and 5*).

Suggested oils (always dilute): Jasmine, Olibanum Essential Oil, Frankincense Essential Oil, Myrrh Essential Oil and Lavandula officinalis Essential Oil

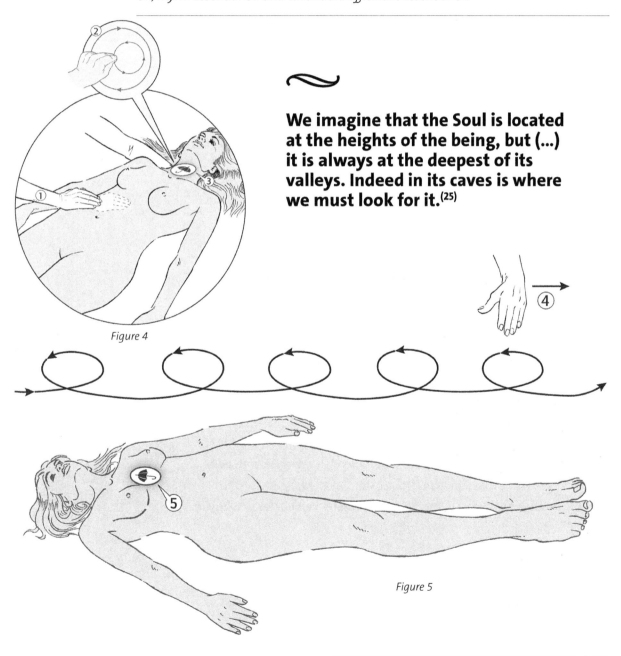

We imagine that the Soul is located at the heights of the being, but (...) it is always at the deepest of its valleys. Indeed in its caves is where we must look for it.[25]

Figure 4

Figure 5

15) Multiple sclerosis

Although obviously not known as such by the ancient therapists, this disease, by its symptoms, had attracted their attention to the point that they had established a healing protocol to at least slow the progression of the disease.

* See p. 147.

In modern terms, multiple sclerosis, whose origin remains mysterious, is defined as a chronic autoimmune neurological disease that attacks the central nervous system. Studies have indicated that it causes a loss of myelin nerve fibers of the brain, spinal cord and optic nerve. The Essenians and the ancient Egyptians believed that this disease was essentially of causal origin, and it referred in most cases to a deep-rooted problem of self-esteem. However, the term "causal" did not and still does not mean "unhealable."

Life is always at the end of life. It replants itself by feeding on its own metamorphoses. [31]

Phase 1: Place your client in a prone position or on his or her side if the prone position is uncomfortable.

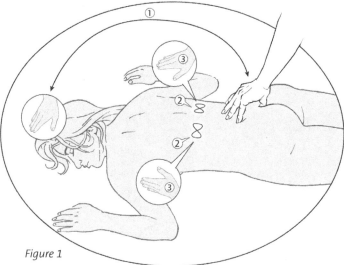

a) Bring along a resonance from the top of the client's skull to the base of the coccyx, no matter the polarity of your hands. Lightly massage the base of the coccyx with your finger in a clockwise direction. Call the Light through you and ask for help *(Figure 1, Landmark 1).*

Figure 1

b) With the help of a little oil, simultaneously energize both adrenal glands by massaging in lemniscates. Meanwhile, call up the image of a moon that gradually becomes a sun before calling for their Archetypes *(Landmark 2).*

c) Place your hand flat on the top of each of the client's kidneys to create an energetic belt on his back. You can also accomplish this gesture on the etheric area of the kidneys without physical contact *(Landmark 3).*

Figure 2

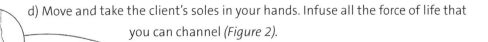

d) Move and take the client's soles in your hands. Infuse all the force of life that you can channel (*Figure 2*).

e) With the Method of the Unified Three Fingers or the Dropper, offer the Wave of Healing to the entire medullar area. During this time, visualize the flame of a candle (*Figure 3, Landmark 4*).

f) Place both your hands flat close by to the cardiac chakra. You could do this on the etheric field of this area (*Landmark 5*).

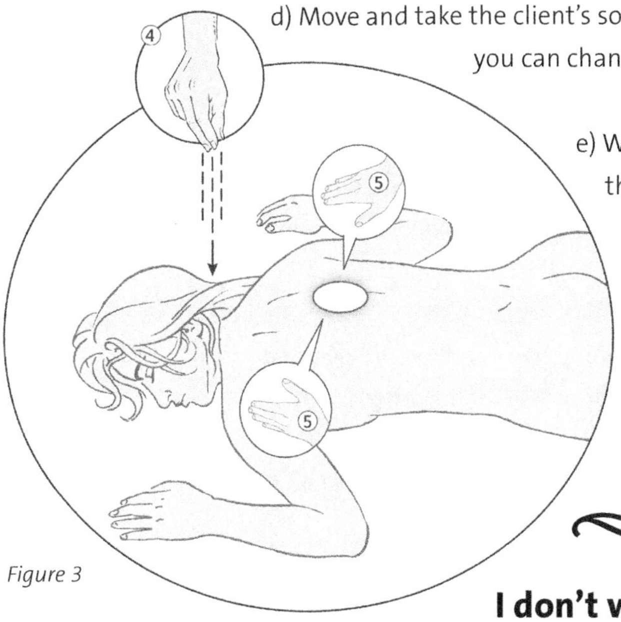

Figure 3

I don't want to honor the wind, but the Power that makes it rise. I don't want to bow down the fire anymore, but bless the Breath of life that makes it be of what to be. I don't want to serve the stone anymore, but love the Flame that makes it matrix. I don't want to worship water anymore but drink the Celestial Earth that makes it the gift of its transparency.[32]

Phase 2: Place your client in the supine position.

g) Harmonize the client's laryngeal chakra using The Method of the Umbrella while visualizing a stream of running water (*Figure 4, Landmark 6*).

h) Using one or two fingers, massage the two secondary chakras of the shoulders vigorously in a clockwise direction (*Landmark 7*).

i) After applying some oil, execute a series of lemniscastes from the fifth to the second chakras. Do two or three round trips from top to bottom and from bottom to top (*Landmark 8*).

j) Use the method of the United Three Fingers or the Dropper at the level of the frontal chakra (*Landmark 9*).

k) Harmonize the client's cardiac chakra in the traditional manner while internally visualizing an intense flame (*Landmark 10*).

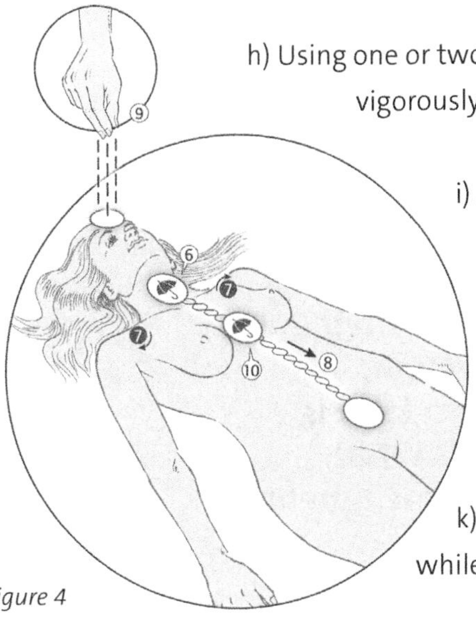

Figure 4

16) PROSTATITIS

a) Start by creating resonance on the frontal chakra of your client by laying your supportive hand on it and placing the United Three Fingers of your active hand. Given the intimate area that these three fingers will treat, namely the perineum, first inform your client and obtain his agreement to avoid any misunderstanding. This resonance setting is followed by solar circulation *(Landmark 1)*.

b) Meanwhile, your unified three fingers of your active hand remain directed toward the perineum, and you move your supportive hand and place it, and the unified three fingers, at the base of the pubis bone of your client. Emit the wave of healing simultaneously through the tips of the fingers of both hands. The goal is to converge the two beams toward the prostate *(Landmark 2)*.

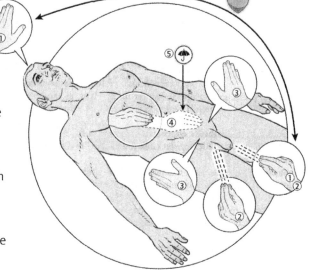

c) Place both your hands flat bottom to top on each of the ureters *(Landmark 3)*.

d) Internalize some more, and then release the astral counterpart of your active hand and let it gently penetrate the client's entire etheric bladder-prostate field. Infuse all with the Light *(Landmark 4)*.

e) Lastly, rebalance the second chakra using the Method of the Umbrella *(Landmark 5)*.

Suggested oils (always dilute): "Masculine Presence", "Chakra 6", Rose of Damascus Essential Oil, White or Yellow Sandalwood Essential Oil, and Neroli Essential Oil

---

Don't curse the narrowness of the doors you are asked to go through. A hardship is always a sign that the Divine is taking care of you. If It plows the field of your soul, It is because It intends to sow something. When a land is tilled, the weed has its roots upside down. This is what hurts. So don't see your suffering as a curse or a punishment but as a preparation.[33]

17) Addiction

This treatment is intended to help people addicted to toxic substances—drugs, tobacco or alcohol—to develop clearer views of their lives and to spark them into reversing their destructive behavior. During a crisis and the development of a comprehensive, long-term treatment plan, apply this treatment about three to four times a week.

In the case of any addiction, the frontal chakra is particularly disorganized.

a) Apply The Method of the Umbrella at the level of the client's sixth chakra *(Figure 1, Landmark 1).*

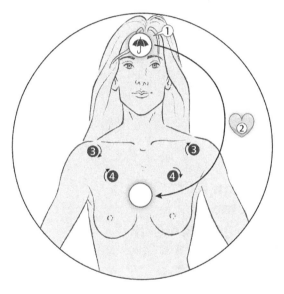

b) Bring resonance to this chakra through the cardiac chakra by Solar Circulation *(Landmark 2).*

c) Using one or two fingers, firmly massage the secondary chakras of both the client's shoulders in a clockwise motion *(Landmark 3).*

d) Do the same at the level of the subchakras located in the middle of the chest, on each side of the sternum *(Landmark 4).*

e) Ask your client to turn to the other side, and create resonance using Solar Circulation in the area of the coccyx and the posterior face of the sixth chakra. Place the active hand on this chakra *(Figure 2, Landmark 5).*

While this treatment certainly is dynamic when we consider the amount of pressure it requires, it focuses on invigorating and supporting the will of the client, and it must occur in conjunction with deep psychotherapy.

Suggested oils (always dilute): "Lucidity", "Addiction", Rose of Damascus Essential Oil, Frankincense Essential Oil , Jasmine and peppermint Essential Oils (diluted)

~

**It is not the body to be exceeded;
this is the soul in the successive layers
of its blindness and its rigid habits
because the roots of a tree are in all
respects like its branches.**

**The trunk, the soul, is similar to an axis
of ascension; don't see in it the major
expression of the tree; it is not the beginning
nor the completion, only an intermediate
from where Heaven and Earth embrace...
which is finished by making a fire.[34]**

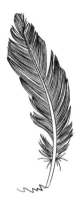

TENTH PART

The Feminine Treatments

For practical reasons, we thought it useful to have a chapter dedicated to the treatments specifically for women. As you will notice, some treatments are curative and others more preventive, while some are simply to help during pregnancy.

If you believe it seems wise, logical and good that a child is born after the exact time in the womb of a mother, why don't you accept that a soul needs its right time to recognize itself?[37]

1) Irregular menstrual cycles

This treatment is designed to help women who suffer from irregular menstrual cycles. It aims to regulate both the amount and duration of the flow through precise work at the level of the chakras.

a) First, create resonance in the second and sixth chakras using Solar Circulation *(Figure 1, Landmark 1)*.

b) Create an Etheric Incision from the right ovary to the left ovary. This incision ideally should be shaped slightly like a circle arc. When the etheric body is open, infuse with your United Three Fingers all the Light possible. Close the incision and seal it *(Landmark 2)*.

c) Simultaneously place the United Three Fingers of your supportive hand (S) on the right ovary and the United Three Fingers of your active hand (A) on the frontal chakra. Let Light act through you *(Landmarks 3S and 3A)*.

d) In the same state of mind, place your supportive hand flat on the right ovary and, simultaneously, direct a beam of the United Three Fingers of your active hand on the solar chakra. Take all the time necessary to infuse Light *(Landmarks 4S and 4A)*.

e) Do the same with the other ovary. Place the tips of your United Three Fingers of your supportive hand (left ovary) and at the same time focus the beam of the three fingers of your active hand on the sixth chakra *(Figure 2, Landmarks 5S and 5A)*.

f) While lying your supportive hand flat on the left ovary, direct the beam of your active hand toward the third chakra *(Landmarks 6S and 6A)*.

g) Practice now, always in great awareness, a big Etheric Incision on the front of the body from the fifth chakra to the second. Open the etheric tissues and infuse the wave of healing with the light brush *(Landmarks 7 and 8)*.

h) Lastly, balance the fifth, fourth and second chakras using the Umbrella Method (Landmarks 9, 10 and 11).

   Don't forget to carefully close and smooth the etheric wound that was created.

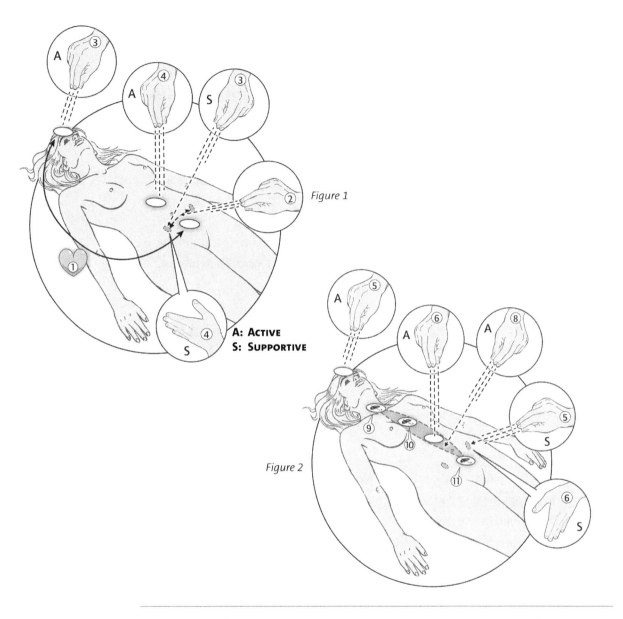

Figure 1

Figure 2

A: Active
S: Supportive

Suggested oils (always dilute): "Feminine Presence", "Lucidity", "Chakra 6", Rose of Damascus Essential Oil, Spruce Hemlock Essential Oil, and Myrrh Essential Oil.

Note: By her subtle physiological nature, woman captures in abundance the multiple forms of the etheric circulation of the planet, much more than man. Her etheric body retransmits various information to the blood. It exists within her "safety valve," which gives rise to the phenomenon of the menstrual cycles. The major centers concerned with these cycles are the sixth and the second chakras. The second dilates, leading the peripheral nadis and the ovaries to dilate themselves and fill up with an etheric energy, leading to ovulation. Abnormalities result from a disruption of this system at a point where it meets another.

2) CIRCULATORY PROBLEMS OF THE LEGS

Pregnant women frequently have circulatory problems in their legs. However, this treatment is suitable not only for pregnant women but for all women having circulatory problems in their legs. It is particularly suitable if the client feels heaviness or mild pains in the pelvis, in the groin folds and along the legs.

For the sake of clarity, our illustration mentions only the left side of the body. However, the treatment should also be applied to the right side. The two sides can be treated simultaneously if the fluidity appeals to the movements and consciousness of the therapist.

a) Start by harmonizing the second then the third chakra in the traditional manner. After this harmonization, consider bringing resonance through Solar Circulation *(Landmarks 1 and 2).*

b) With one or two fingers, massage the secondary chakra of the last floating rib using small lemniscates *(Landmark 3).*

c) Do the same at the point of the iliac crest, and then extend your lemniscates along the nadis leading to the energetic point of the groin *(Landmarks 4 and 5).*

d) From the point of the groin, go down along the major nadi of the leg by always moving with small strokes in lemniscates until the point located at mid-height and behind of the calf. On the way, firmly massage the point at mid-height of the leg and the popliteal fossa *(Landmarks 5, 6, 7 and 8).*

Note: It is imperative to use an oil for this treatment.

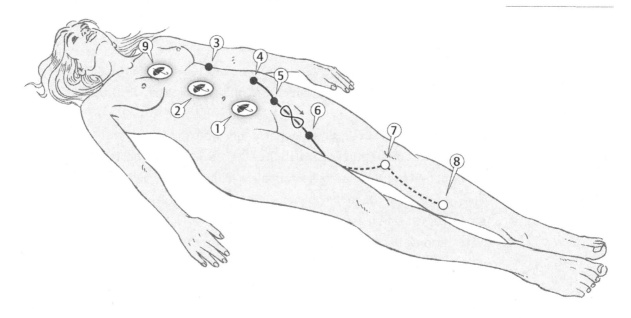

Note: These small massage movements in lemniscates must be sustained. To be more active cleaning the etheric waste, each path between two points must be executed from top to bottom then bottom to top several times.

e) Finish by rebalancing the cardiac chakra in the traditional manner (Landmark 9).

Note: The movements recommended in lemniscates here are not given as a simple physical massage but are infused with love. They require a "channeling" state of Light from the therapist as part of a sacred process. Such treatment needs to be repeated regularly to avoid dirtying of the nadis of the legs and the pelvis, which frequent occurs during pregnancy.

3) THE ENERGETIC DISORDERS OF THE PREGNANT WOMAN

As its name suggests, this simple treatment is aimed at various energetic disorders generated by pregnancy. It also can prevent these disorders from developing. Ideally, it should be practiced once a week, especially concerning the Etheric Incision applied to the folds of the groin and armpits. These four areas are where etheric snags stagnate and often develop significant mass.

a) First, put in resonance the second and third chakras using Solar Circulation *(Landmark 1).*

b) Repeat it for the fifth and sixth chakras (Landmark 2).

c) Create an Etheric Incision on each armpit and each fold of the groin. Once you have made these subtle openings, use either the method of the United Three Fingers as a brush or the dropper (Landmark 3, 4, 5 and 6).

d) Don't forget to reseal each opening each time you finish your touch with the application of small lemniscates on the incised area. You could create these lemniscates two ways: directly on the skin after applying some oil or in the etheric body of the incised area.

Suggested oils (always use in small quantities and dilute during pregnancy): "Welcome", "Revealing", Rose of Damascus Essential oil, and Lavandula officinalis Lavender Essential Oil.

4) MISCARRIAGES AND ABORTIONS

Although miscarriages and abortions obviously have different causes, the energetic disruptions left on the subtle bodies share similarities. The Essenian and Egyptian therapists therefore addressed them in the same way to help the feminine organism to restore its balance.

The global objective is to apply an energetic bandage promoting healing of the mental, emotional and etheric wounds, which never fail to be created in such painful circumstances. It goes without saying that the delicacy, the listening, the expertise and the love of the therapist are solicited here in their maximum.

a) Start by applying Solar Circulation to the second and sixth chakras. Place your active (A) hand on the sixth chakra and your supporting (S) hand on the second chakra *(Figure 1, Landmark 1)*.

b) With the United Three Fingers like a brush of your active hand, move down very slowly from the frontal chakra along the median to finally reach the second chakra, where your supportive hand is located. It is important that you visualize, perceive internally, draw or take a stream of Light down during your descent of the median *(Landmark 2)*.

c) Once you arrive at the second chakra, spread the United Three Fingers of your active hand to place your hand flat close by the supportive hand, which you have kept still since the beginning of the treatment. You could choose to hold both hands flat in the etheric area of your client. Infuse all the Light possible *(Landmark 3)*.

d) Unify the three fingers of your active hand once more and draw with their beam an Operative Field on the lower abdomen. Your supportive hand can leave the second chakra during this time *(Landmark 4)*.

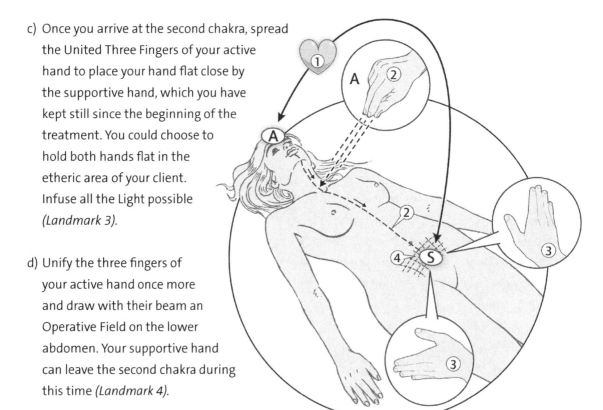

Figure 1

e) Create a big Etheric Incision horizontally on the area that has been vibrationally disinfected. Open the subtle wound with your second hand and immediately infuse it with the wave of healing using the traditional method of the three fingers of your active hand. The beam emitted will ideally be emerald green or golden white *(Figure 2, Landmarks 5 and 6)*.

f) Slowly bring your three fingers closer to the etheric opening. Open your hand and place it on your client's skin. Internalize and start to extract your astral hand from your physical hand according to the method described previously, and then let your astral hand make energetic contact with the uterus. If you feel or know that the physical contact of your hand on the skin can make her uncomfortable or upset her, do the same but remain in the etheric space of your client *(Landmark 7)*.

g) Delicately return your astral hand to yourself before carefully closing and smoothing the etheric wound.

h) Put in resonance the second and third chakras and then the second and fourth chakras through the Solar Method *(Landmarks 8 and 9)*.

A prayer of thanks to the Divine, to the Sacred of Life will be particularly welcome.

Suggested oils (always dilute): "Repairing Balm", Jasmine Essential Oil, "Presence Feminine", Rose of Damascus Essential Oil, Myrrh Essential oil, and Frankincense Essential Oil.

**Don't save anything in you
Call the Force of Life and
redistribute It!
Call Love and multiply It!
Move down Peace,
And spread It like a water
infiltrating everywhere.**[36]

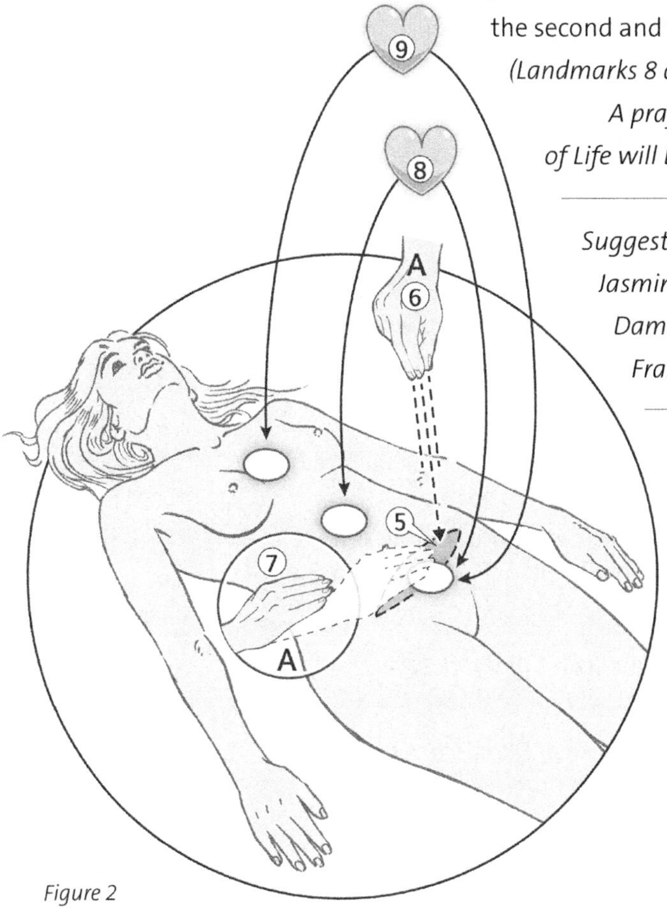

Figure 2

5) Pre-Menopause and Menopause

a) First, physically and etherically, draw the Archetype of the moon–solar star or the Egyptian key–cross of life on the client's forehead on the front chakra of the forehead six times.[16] Ideally, apply an essential oil of rose or jasmine to the center of this chakra prior to drawing the symbols *(Landmark 1)*.

b) Position yourself at your client's head and slowly move both your hands to the person's temples. After establishing either physical or etheric contact with the client, visualize a green wave moving from each of your hands to the heart of the frontal chakra *(Landmark 2)*.

c) Feel this green wave moving slowly down along the whole body from the frontal chakra to the second chakra *(Landmark 3)*.

d) Place your hands on each ovary and, from them, send an orange luminous beam toward the second chakra *(Landmark 4)*.

e) Place your active hand in the zone of radiance of the second chakra and try to feel its radiance. It must have intensified, as you had directed an orange healing wave toward it. Observe the beam emitted closely until you feel a true luminous spherical presence in the palm of your hand. Apply this luminous presence in the vibrational space of your client's uterus *(Figure 2, Landmarks 5, 6 and 7)*.

f) Internalize yourself more, and then detach your astral active hand—the one that has the sphere of Light—and slide it carefully and respectfully into the subtle counterpart of the uterus. It is not necessary to create an Etheric Incision beforehand *(Landmark 8)*.

g) Detach your astral hand from the uterus and reharmonize the second chakra using the traditional Method of the Umbrella *(Landmark 9)*.

h) Put in resonance the second and fifth chakras *(Landmark 10)*.

Suggested oils (always dilute): "Feminine Presence", Rose of Damascus Essential Oil and Myrrh Essential Oil.

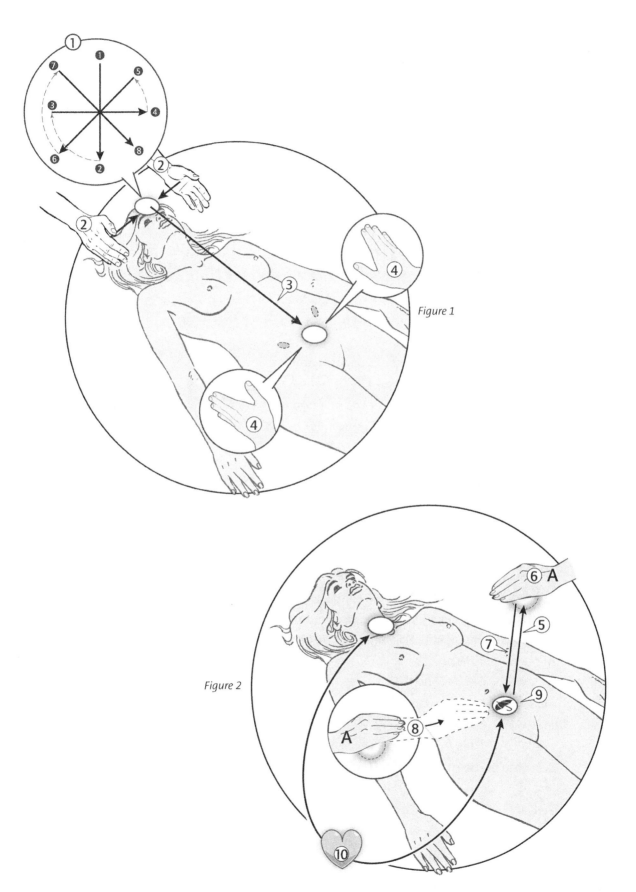

Figure 1

Figure 2

6) INFERTILITY

*See p. 123.

This treatment requires substantial work. It requires, on one hand, to be practiced at least once a week for a minimum of a month, and on the other hand, to be preceded by the treatment of the Thoughts-Forms. Most women who experience difficulty conceiving or whose infertility seems an inarguable fact develop one or multiple Thoughts-Forms of self-depreciation or guilt related to this problem. Thus, while considering the problem at the physiological level, the ancient therapists also addressed it at the mental level, or the causal level.

Emphasize, once again, that in their eyes "causal" didn't mean in any way "inescapable."

In parallel to the recommended work here, treatment of the Archetypes—as indicated in the advanced practices section—may prove useful.

Figure 1

a) Start with the treatment of the Thoughts-Forms.*

b) Place yourself at your client's feet and massage the middle of the sole of her left foot using long strokes and moving in a clockwise direction. For this, use a grounding oil *(Figure 1)*.

c) Place yourself on the side of your client according to the polarity of your hands, at the level of her legs. Take the heel of her left foot with your active hand and slide your supportive hand under her left knee. Internalize and perceive the entire area between the heel and the knee as infused with Light. Put an energetic "surge" into it in a loving way, without imposing any direction on the circulation of the currents *(Figure 2)*.

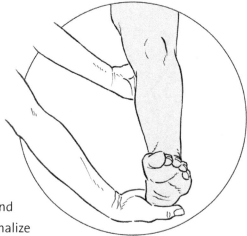

Figure 2

d) Place your supportive hand on your client's groin and your active hand under her knee, so you go up one "floor" on her leg. Observe the same mindset described previously *(Figure 3)*.

e) Repeat these steps on the right leg.
Note that you could start this treatment on the right leg and then continue on the left leg.

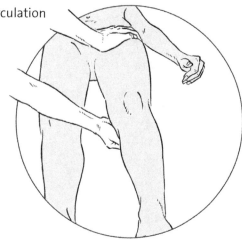

Figure 3

f) Create an Etheric Incision in the traditional way on each of the two ovaries, one after another *(Figure 4, Landmark 1)*.

g) Simultaneously place the United Three Fingers of each of your hands above the two etheric wounds and then open them. Center yourself and practice Solar Circulation. Once it reaches your heart, the wave of healing will move toward the right ovary, passing by your right arm. Maintain this energetic loop for a while *(Landmark 2)*.

h) After sealing the two etheric openings of the ovaries, place your active hand flat on the corresponding area of the uterus of your client, and slide it progressively within your astral hand. Focus on delicacy *(Landmark 3)*.

i) Reharmonize the second chakra in the traditional way *(Landmark 4)*.

j) Create resonance on this chakra using Solar Circulation with the laryngeal chakra then the frontal chakra.

Suggested oils (always dilute): "Heart", "Feminine Presence", Rrose of Damascus Essential Oil and Myrrh Essential Oil

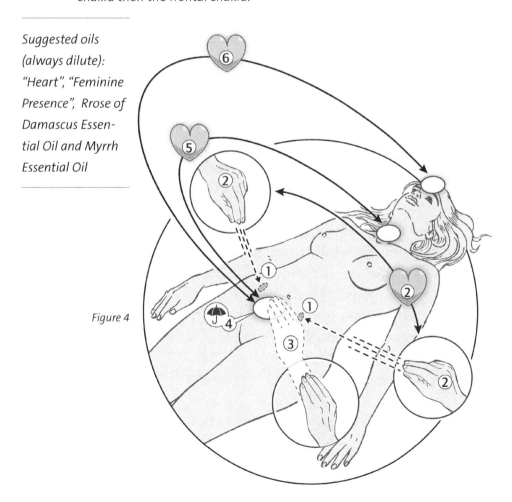

Figure 4

7) BREAST CANCER

Never say that this treatment will cure breast cancer—it would be dangerous for a woman to rely only on this treatment if she were diagnosed with this disease. However, the treatment described here can be a significant help in the treatment of such a cancer. It aims to clean and fluidize the energetic relationships along the nadis, which are especially challenged in this case.

This treatment relates the infected breast to the opposite ovary. There is always a "crossed" energetic connection between a breast and an ovary, even in the case of a healthy organism. It is therefore a cleaning and supportive treatment, which can, in this sense, promote the restoration of the organism. Our example presupposes a cancer of the right breast.

Suggested oils (always dilute): "Revealing", "Feminine Presence", Rose of Damascus Essential Oil, Spruce Hemlock Essential Oil and Nard Essential Oil.

a) With an oil, on the internal face of the arm, start tracing with your finger a series of small lemniscates along the nadis, which unify the secondary chakra to the wrist of the concerned arm and the point located in the armpit. You can repeat this cleaning and strengthening movement two or three times in a row.

At each point of energetic force, do a little counterclockwise massage. This will allow the dispersion of the etheric snags *(Landmark 1)*.

b) By Etheric Palpation, attempt to locate the nadis that unify the end of the armpit with the extremity of the breast. Make this nadis dynamic like you have done for the arm using small lemniscates *(Landmark 2)*.

c) Do the same by following the path of the nadis that unifies the sub-chakra of the shoulder with the extremity of the breast *(Landmark 3)*.

d) Create resonance from the point of the secondary chakra of the armpit to the opposite ovary of the treated breast using Solar Circulation. Use the Unified Three Fingers of each hand, regardless of the polarity of the hand in contact with the ovary: Solar Circulation is dominant *(Landmark 4)*.

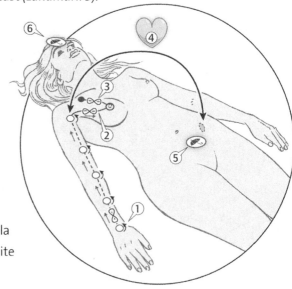

e) Harmonize using The Method of the Umbrella the second and sixth chakras by calling a white Light in both cases *(Landmarks 5 and 6)*.

8) Breast nodules

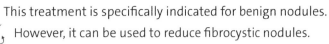

This treatment is specifically indicated for benign nodules. However, it can be used to reduce fibrocystic nodules.

a) Start with one or two fingers by gently massaging the point located at the crook of the client's elbow, on the side of the affected breast, in a counterclockwise direction. With the same two fingers, go up by small lemniscates along the nadis, which brings you to the energetic point of the armpit. Massage it counterclockwise as well *(Landmark 1)*.

b) There are five important energy points that lie across the circumference of the breast. Massage them gently, always clockwise and moving from the outside of the body toward the inner face of the breast *(Landmark 2)*.

c) Create five small etheric incisions very delicately from the nipple toward each of these points. Don't open these incisions but infuse the Wave of Healing on each of their paths by using the Method of the United Three Fingers as a brush or a dropper. Smooth each of these incisions in the ether to seal them *(Landmark 3)*.

d) The extremity of a breast naturally emits a little luminous gushing over a distance of a few centimeters. In the case of nodules, this gushing is cluttered with etheric snags. From the end of the three united fingers of your active hand, try to make energetic contact with this gushing. As soon as you "grasp" it, "magnetize" it with your Three Fingers by moving away from the extremity of the breast with a counterclockwise movement as energetically as possible. Repeat this gesture many times, and then bring your active hand over the flame of a candle *(Landmarks 4 and 5)*.

e) Gently massage the subchakra of the shoulder of the treated breast in a clockwise direction *(Landmark 6)*.

Suggested oils (always dilute): Rose of Damascus Essential Oil and Nard Essential Oil.

f) Successively reharmonize the sixth and the fourth chakras using the Method of the Umbrella *(Landmarks 7 and 8)*.

Insist on the reharmonization of the cardiac chakra because most of the nodules of the breast have an affective origin and frequently point to low self-esteem.

The Divine is All.

You can not cut It away from your life,
neither make It as a simple element
of your inner life, an element that
we remember only when everything
goes wrong.

It is All because It is Life and you
are immerged into It as It is within you.

So you can leave everything except Its
footprints and Its path in you.[37]

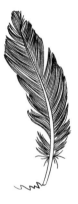

ELEVENTH PART

The Advanced Practices

The treatments we present here are deemed advanced because they require the implementation of advanced skills by students who are familiar with the background and practices of the Essenian and Egyptian therapies discussed thus far. It means students are not only comfortable with the technical aspects of the treatments, which allows them to work with fluidity, but also have developed the mindset required and the ability to gauge the "energetic feeling" of the bodies and souls they treat.

In other words, these therapies require that therapists refine their receptive capacity and their potential of transmission and emission. Therefore, this is their loving way of listening to the other, which is crucial in the application of the techniques described in this chapter. Similarly, the therapist's connection with the Presence of the Divine will be especially necessary. This connection is of course an invitation to come closer to the state of Advaita, that of Unity in the All, the joyful promise of a great expansion of the consciousness.

1) THE LANGUAGE OF THE VERTEBRAE

The basic principles of this technique were revealed at the temple of Kom Ombo in Egypt and were restructured a second time in the city of Akhetaton before being refined a final time between the walls of the Essenian monastery of Krmel.

This is not a healing technique in the strict sense but rather a method of evaluating the nature of the inner disorders affecting a client. Founded on a long observation of the human being combined with a keen sense of synthesis, it is based on the fact that each vertebra of the human body is closely related to an expression of the being, all at once physical, emotional, mental and spiritual. Any vertebra, according its location and its function, can translate a need, a call, a fear, a lack or an excess.

It is essential that the therapist obtain the permission of the client before performing a "reading." This treatment is justified and successful only if clients feel the need to move forward with their lives and to "work on [their] interior foundations" to improve their overall health through improved relationships with themselves, others and Life in general. The information the therapist provides after interpreting the language of the vertebrae can be valuable material for personal advancement while halting the development of possible pathologies.

To ensure the effectiveness and preciseness of the treatment, this method requires mastery of Etheric Palpation, particularly on the dorsal axis.

It is imperative that your client is in the prone position—or at least on his or her side—to facilitate access to the radiance of the entire dorsal axis.

a) Slowly palpate the etheric spine with the help of the most sensitive area of your active hand. Traditionally, it was suggested to practice this palpation from bottom to top, but nothing suggests that this direction is mandatory. What is imperative is the attention you give to any noticeable perceptions along the backbone. Apply yourself to noticing the areas that seem to be expressing fragility, blockage or disharmony.

b) After memorizing the affected areas following the comprehensive identification you made, proceed with greater precision. If you found several, place your supportive hand on the first area that caught your attention. Simultaneously, slowly place your active hand—fingers or wrist—on a detailed map of the vertebrae related to the initial marked area. Focus all your consciousness on this hand.

When your active hand is in contact with the disharmonious vertebra on the map, it will send you a signal, a sensation that may be difficult to express but revealing. Identify this vertebra and refer to the map of interpretation provided in this book.

In summary, if you noted a dissonance or a possible blockage at, for example, the level of the lumbar vertebrae during the first Etheric Palpation, the refined approach will allow you to use two hands—one on the lumbar vertebrae and the other, the active one, on the map—to determine precisely which lumbar vertebra must be considered. If it is located at about L4, for instance, and you have done your work well, you can deduce by consulting the table that it is likely to be a problem regarding your client's "fear of the future."

Repeat the process for all the vertebral areas that caught your attention.

Listening to your client allows them to reflect on matters, and after this, the information imparted by the their vertebrae will be as important to him or her as it is to you. In your role of therapist, it will improve your understanding of the origin of disorders or fragilities that require your help.

Happiness is a state of offering in which the purest part of your being already constantly bathes, a state that never generates lack or exhaustion.

It is a state of abundance of the heart.

This state of abundance is infinite because (...) the one who lets it be revealed within him has nothing to defend because he doesn't appropriate anything.

And he doesn't appropriate anything by only the fact that he feels and knows being present in everything, sharing everything with everything.[38]

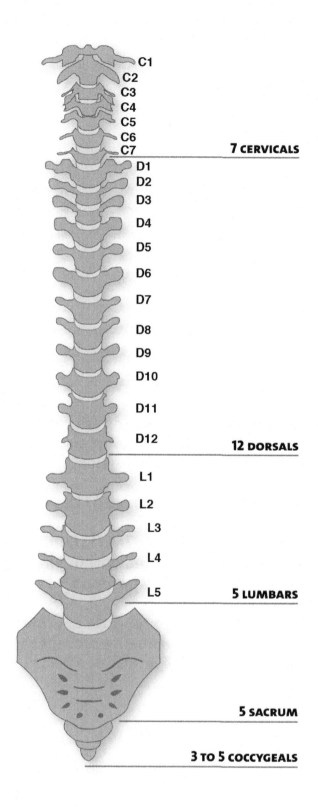

C1
C2
C3
C4
C5
C6
C7

D1
D2
D3
D4
D5
D6
D7
D8
D9
D10
D11
D12

L1
L2
L3
L4
L5

7 CERVICALS

12 DORSALS

5 LUMBARS

5 SACRUM

3 TO 5 COCCYGEALS

TABLE OF INTERPRETATION OF THE LANGUAGE OF THE VERTEBRAE

Roots	Coccyx	Difficulties of incarnation
Fears	Sacrum	General insecurity
	Five lumbar vertebrae	L5: Need to clear the past L4: Fear of the future L3: Fear of disease L2: Confusion, lack of perspective facing life L1: Lack of assertiveness
"Points of Ego"	The 12 dorsal vertebrae	D12: Important and global difficulty to master the ego D11: Necessity to master recurring emotions D10: Need for freedom of expression D9: Difficult confrontation with Matter D8: Necessity to purify the mind D7: Tendency to arrogance D6: Excessive carnal appetites D5: Excessive need to control others D4: Lack of self-confidence D3: Excessive dispersion D2: Need to find an ideal D1: Need for an elevating experience, to take stock of a situation
Relationship with Spirit	The seven cervical vertebrae	C7: Need to look beyond the material world C6: Fear of a judgment, conviction, verdict C5: Difficult confrontation with duality C4: Need to rebel C3: Nostalgia, weariness of Light C2: Awakening latent or manifestation of a deep memory C1: Desperate need of equity; wounded due to injustice

2) The therapy of the Archetypes

For most of us, it is important to recognize that the notion of archetype is rather vague. We view "archetype" as a synonym for "symbol." However, an archetype and a symbol differ greatly, like a number and a figure or, in our area of study, the Akasha and the Ether.

In the Divine world, the Archetype is a primal Principle; in other words, it is one of the basic materials directly received from the Spirit creator during the emission of a Wave of Life. It is a Force, a live and conscious Presence that carries within it certain functions of the Divine and their internal developments. These are the developments that we named the symbols. Thus, an Archetype can generate many symbols, each with its specificities depending on the eras, races and periods. As a symbol will tap its breath in the Archetype from which it originates, we can draw the analogy that it corresponds to the world of the Soul, while the Archetype responds to the world of Spirit.

When we refer to an Archetype, we must be aware that we do not address a harmless strength but rather an intelligent Presence directly from the Divine. We invoke what is called a "power" in the best sense of the term.[17]

Consequently, therapists must use the Archetype treatment with great respect and an acute consciousness of the triangular relationship, the importance of which we have already discussed.

During deep work undertaken with a client, it can have a surprising effect. Given the descent of Energy it generates, both in the therapist and the person being healed, this treatment was considered by the Egyptians as part of their secret knowledge.

However, For the sake of simplicity, we do not use the Archetypal designs. Instead, we use their Hebraic counterparts, established by the Essenian insiders to include them in their therapeutic Tradition.

Like the method of vertebrae reading, the process used in the therapy of the Archetypes presupposes an overall healing of will, the client's wish to evolve at all levels of the life journey and not simply scratching the surface of the client's being. Its purpose is to treat the imperfections of the personality as well as the deep weaknesses of the physical organism. Thus, these difficulties should be the subject of an intense and sincere exchange between therapist and client prior to the treatment. In addition, this treatment may follow a reading of the vertebrae to further the work undertaken by conducting a "scouring" supporting the being, body, soul and spirit.

The principle of this treatment is based on the fact that a problem is always connected to a chakra, this chakra corresponds to a symbol and this symbol to an Archetype. The reference grid uses seven geometric figures as a symbol and twenty-two archetypal letters.

a) First of all, ask your client to choose his or her points of concern on the list of twenty-one descriptions plus the one listed on the two attached tables. The client must choose no more than three. Note these points, and have your client lie down on his or her back or stomach, which is preferred.

b) Start with the first problem identified by your client. On the table, find how it corresponds to a chakra, then draw the associated geometric figure above this chakra in your client's etheric, emotional or mental aura, as the case may be. You must trace this figure the number of times indicated (between 1 and 9). This practice allows a vibrational door to open in the Invisible, facilitating access to an Archetype.

c) Once finished, draw the corresponding Archetype of the chakra that has been treated on your client's skin no more than three times. Do this in absolute awareness of a connection with the Divine, and follow with intense meditation. *(See our table for the drawing of the Archetype.)*

d) Move to the treatment of the second problem, still referring to the reference grid.

Example: If your client recognizes a problem of possessiveness, the need to control, the person must be treated at the level of the sixth chakra (Ajna). You draw two vertical parallel lines six times in the etheric aura of this chakra, and then, three times, the Archetype corresponding to the Hebraic letter "Vau" on the skin at the location of the same chakra.

---

e) Ideally, always finish this type of treatment with a treatment of your client's eighth chakra, located in the embryonic principle about 50 centimeters (20 inches) above the body. This acts as the seal of closure of the sacred act that has been carried out. Draw the geometric symbol of the moon and the sun, as illustrated in the table, eight times in the vibrational space of the eighth chakra, Tekla. Next, draw the Archetypal letter corresponding to "Tau" three times at the top of your client's skull.

All those who are aware of the Consciousness are united by golden threads beyond the Ages. This is the logic of this frame by which they live, support and is important to them. Each gathers the love and the wisdom of their predecessors and offers his own gifts to those who are following along the great ladder of the Plan.[39]

#	Problem Detected	Chakra Concerned	Symbol	Times	Level of Aura	Body Archetype	Times	Letter	Letter Name
1	Rooting, difficulty being in the everyday	1st (Muladhara)	■	1	Etheric	✕	3	A	Aleph
2	Excessive sense of belonging bloodline law primary sexuality	2nd (Svadishatana)	▶	2	Etheric	⌐	3	B	Beth
3	Instability, irritability, need to wander, polarization on the physical	3rd (Manipura)	✚	3	Etheric	⌐	3	G	Gimel
4	Cardiac difficulties of all kinds	4th (Anahata)	●	4	Etheric	⌐	3	D	Daleth
5	Breathing problems of all kinds	5th (Vishuddha)	◀	5	Etheric	⌐	3	E	Hé
6	Possessiveness, need to count or control	6th (Ajna)	‖	6	Etheric	⌐	3	V	Vau
7	Unhealthy need to dominate, to impose	7th (Sahasrara)	•	7	Etheric	⌐	3	Z	Zain
8	Sickly terrorism	1st (Muladhara)	■	8	Emotional	⌐	4	H	is
9	Excessive pursuit of all carnal appetites	2nd (Svadishtana)	▶	9	Emotional	⌐	3	Th	Teth
10	Need to control followers to value themselves	3rd (Manipura)	✚	1	Emotional	⌐	3	J	Jod
11	Unhealthy need for love or attention	4th (Anahata)	●	2	Emotional	⌐	3	K	Caph

#	Problem Detected	Chakra Concerned	Symbol	Times	Level of Aura	Body Archetype	Times	Letter	Letter Name
12	Thoughtless, often destructive speech	5th (Vishuddha)	◀	3	Emotional	ל	3	L	Lamed
13	Excessive naivety, difficulty with discernment	6th (Ajna)	☰	4	Emotional	ם	3	L	Lamed
14	Personality too analytic, thinks he or she understands and is master of all	7th (Sahadishtana)	•	5	Emotional	נ	3	N	Nuth
15	Mental desire to elevate everyday matters	1st (Muldhara)	■	6	Mental	ס	3	S	Semek
16	Sex is perceived as a tool of manipulation	2nd (Svadishtana)	▶	7	Mental	ע	3	O	Ayn
17	Problems of hyperactivity of the mind, cerebral bulimia	3rd (Manipura)	✚	8	Mental	פ	3	P	Phé
18	Constant need to persuade or teach	4th (Anahata)	●	9	Mental	צ	3	TS	Tsadé
19	Pride pushing to imitate the Master or the creator	5th (Vishudha)	◀	1	Mental	ק	3	Q	Quef
20	Regular use of lies to dominate, mythomania	6th (Ajna)	☰	2	Mental	ר	3	R	Resh
21	Imperious need for power, misguided in the illusion of domination	7th (Sahasrara)	•	3	Mental	ש	3	Sch	Schin
22	TEKLA	8th	○	8	Supra-Consciousness	ת	3	T	Teu

3) THE HEALING OF THE PETALS

Like the methods described previously in this chapter, this method was reserved for the most advanced therapists in the Essenian fraternity. In addition, this method was used on people who were not necessarily physically ill but who wanted to increase their spiritual awareness. We thus strongly advise students in energy therapies to practice this method together.

Again, this method, while influencing behavioral patterns or latent capabilities, acts by repercussion on organs and functions. It consists of two phases. The first phase is the so-called phase of assessment. It is best to take a break between the phase of assessment and the phase of treatment. This break can actually be used to discuss what appeared during the analysis of the chakras and their petals because this practice is based on the principle that each petal of each chakra carries precise information. Each petal has been numbered for technical reasons. As you can see, in the reference system, each chakra is associated with an Archetype in its Aramean expression and not a Hebraic letter. Further, it is linked to a color and a sound.

Phase 1: The assessment

a) Place yourself at your client's head and delicately touch your forehead to the top of the client's head and place your hands on the person's shoulders. Perform the Method of the Scanner* while focusing on the ladder of the chakras. Memorize which chakra or chakras seem to lack Light or manifest a blockage or an absence of fluidity during the "fighting over" of your consciousness. Exclude the coronal in your analysis.

b) Place yourself on the side of your client while reaching with your active hand and viewing the detailed maps of the problem chakra(s). These maps, chakra by chakra, are provided here.

Start by placing your supportive hand flat on the chakra you first found problematic. With the index finger of your active hand, point consciously and internally, one after the other, at each of the petals of the representation of the chakra concerned on the map. The purpose is to perceive a signal emanating from a petal or petals as your finger points to each in turn. This signal varies from one therapist to another. It can be perceived in the point of the active hand or in the form of cardiac feeling.

Always track the petals in a clockwise direction. Each time a petal emits a signal, note the number and refer to the corresponding indication. This will provide important information about your client. Proceed to the analysis of another petal of the same chakra or another chakra that attracted your attention.

* See p. 73.

Phase 2: The treatment

a) Start by reharmonizing the chakra concerned using the Method of the Umbrella.

b) Unlock the heart of this chakra by drawing in its center, with the Three Fingers United of your active hand, the corresponding Aramean Archetype shown in the illustration provided. Draw this Archetype as many times as indicated (close by its dedicated frame). This unlocking requires a lot of love and awareness.

c) Once the heart of the chakra is open, always with your Three Fingers United, project the basic color corresponding to the whole chakra toward it while keeping in mind the number of the petal previously identified.

d) Close the heart of the chakra by again drawing the Aramean Archetype used to open it the same number of times as when opening it.

e) Finish the treatment with a new harmonization of the chakra using The Method of the Umbrella.

Note: *Upon mastering this practice, while emitting the color and focusing on the number of the petal, mentally repeat the basic sound corresponding to the vibration of the chakra. However, don't do this if you haven't mastered the technique.*

You may find it difficult to project a color while focusing on the petal number. You can overcome this difficulty by projecting the image of the number tinted with the required color toward the heart of the chakra.

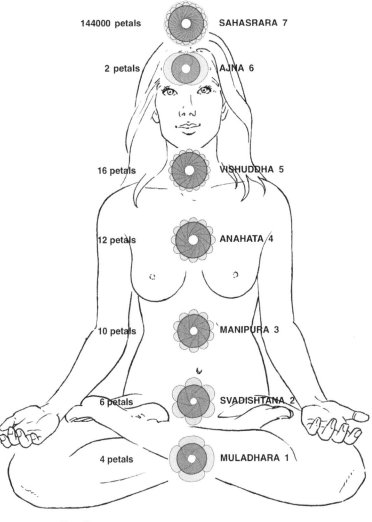

144000 petals — SAHASRARA 7

2 petals — AJNA 6

16 petals — VISHUDDHA 5

12 petals — ANAHATA 4

10 petals — MANIPURA 3

6 petals — SVADISHTANA 2

4 petals — MULADHARA 1

THE SEVEN MAJOR CHAKRAS AND THEIR PETALS

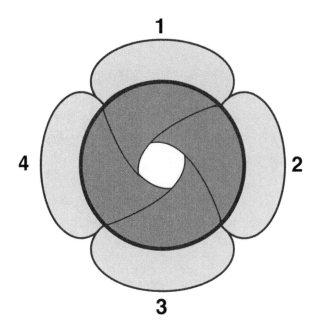

CHAKRA 1
Muladhara

DIRECTOR SOUND
LEM

COLOR
Red

1) Regulation of the ovary or testicles
2) Olfactory capabilities; sexual impulses
3) Sexual force; affirmation level of the ego personality
4) Level to earth and rooting

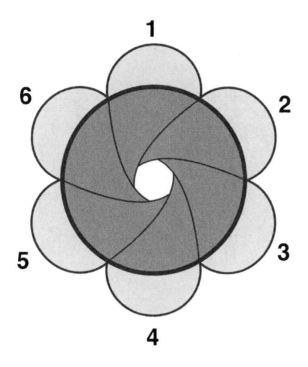

CHAKRA 2
Svadhistana

DIRECTOR SOUND
WAM

COLOR
Orange

1) Adrenals, cellular memorization rate (storage)
2) Gustatory acuity
3) Degree of capability of concretizing
4) Circulation of the Water Element within oneself
5) Skill level to position yourself
6) Physical balance (vertigo or stability)

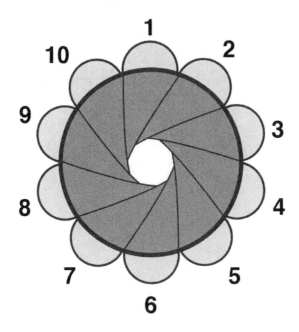

CHAKRA 3
Manipura

DIRECTOR SOUND
REM

COLOR
Yellow

1) Pancreas; potential of the natural defenses
2) Sense of view
3) Control of the evacuation of excrement
4) Fire (physical fore and endurance)
5) Ability to find resources
6) Sense of combativeness
7) Sense of ownership or membership (family, clan, etc.)
8) Need of habits and level of compulsiveness
9) Jealously

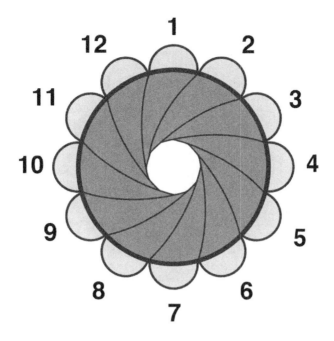

CHAKRA 4
Anahata

DIRECTOR SOUND
YAD

COLOR
Green

1) Thymus: Potential of charisma
2) Sense of touch
3) Air, breathing capabilities
4) Manual ability
5) Empathy, compassion
6) Sense of sharing; level of egoism
7) Artistic capabilities
8) Degree of egocentrism
9) Ability of personal engagement
10) Affective potential; sensitivity
11) Potential of abnegation
12) Sensuality

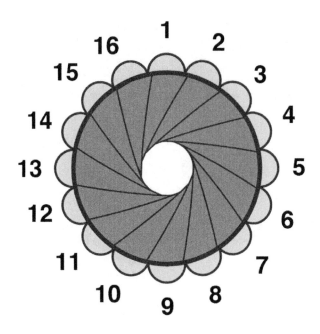

CHAKRA 5
Vishuddha

DIRECTOR SOUND
HEM

COLOR
Light blue

1) Regulation of the thyroid
2) Hearing ability
3) Relationships with Ether;
   subtle food intake
4) Expressive potential (mastery of sound)
5) Sense of personal authority
6) Ability of submission or rebellion
7) Internal generosity rate
8) Level of self-censorship
9) Mastery of the mental activity
   and ability of memorial storage
10) Level of need to control
11) Overall creativity; ingenuity
12) Need to attract
13) Control of desires
14) Sense of equity; intransigence
15) Ability to discern
16) Potential for decision

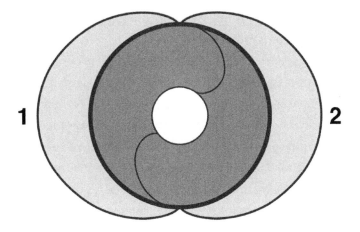

CHAKRA 6
Ajna

DIRECTOR SOUND
AMN

COLOR
Indigo

1) Regulation of the pituitary gland
2) Potential of mastery of supra-sensorial
   perceptions and "mute truths"

Each of these two petals contains forty-eight micro-petals,
making this chakra the leader of the orchestra of the glandular
functions and the subtle capabilities of the being.

4) The Therapy of Surrender

This extremely important therapy refers in particular to the "Geometry of the Awakening" Master Jeshua taught Shlomit (Salomé), one of the first female disciples.[18] Although she did not receive it as such on her person, Shlomit learned the basic principles to teach them in turn. Here is the origin of, from human memory, as well as the elements in which the therapy is grounded.

Like all therapists, the Egyptians and Essenians occasionally encountered cases that resisted all their efforts. Consequently, they developed a treatment method that surpassed their own knowledge and called on the Divine Force to act independently, using their channels to treat the client. As holder of knowledge, they viewed this "letting go" as a last resort, and thus named it the Therapy of Surrender.

Through observation and meditation, they conceived a reference system in which they identified five spheres of life revealed in the incarnated human being:

- The first sphere is defined as a point symbolizing infinity. This point represents the level of connection of the being with the Divine, or at least with his or her own superior consciousness. It involves spiritual maturity.
- The second sphere could symbolize a circle, an image of unity that is self-aware. The ancient therapists viewed this as the area of self-perception, the space of appreciation of events and judgments, cerebral intelligence and common sense.
- The third sphere represents the Two manifesting in the form of a cross. This is the sphere of choices and ability to act; it includes free will and the being's potential to shape his or her life.
- The fourth sphere symbolizes the Three in the form of an equilateral triangle. It translates as the being's area of relationships with all of existence, the overall affective and relational domain, and it allows the expression of cardiac intelligence and the ability to share.
- The fifth sphere represents the Four, symbolized by a square. It expresses the being's degree of incarnation, density, stability and overall solidity.

The Therapy of Surrender that we present here used five major Archetypes: the point, the circle, the cross, the triangle and the square. As we have seen, an Archetype is a direct expression of the Divine Thought in permanent action. Calling upon It means to create or strengthen a bridge of Light that offers all eternity to the Matter in demand. Effective application of this treatment, unsurprisingly, requires three things from the therapist: real compassion, an advanced ability to practice visualization and the total absence of personal challenge.

In this treatment, the expression of "Father, thy will be done" must prevail. This set of Archetypes was implemented in the Houses of Life from the early days of Egypt. It was considered so sacred and powerful in its expression of the incarnated Divine Presence that we should draw it on sand or on the human body.

a) Start by drawing on yourself, with precision and awareness, the global Archetype of the human being as indicated below:

b) Next, draw this same Archetype on the chest of your client, who should be lying down. If possible, use an oil that promotes openness of consciousness.

c) Place the palm of your active hand flat on the cardiac chakra of your client, and then gradually let the double astral aspect of this hand penetrate the center of the rib cage. If the client feels discomfort and experiences the sensation of suffocating, slightly and slowly move your astral hand toward the diaphragm, or third chakra. Place your astral hand longitudinally to the body and from bottom to top.

d) The moment has now come for you to enter an even greater state of internalization. With your hand still discorporate in the organism of your client, visualize the Archetype of the square. It could be that this square spontaneously appears to you in red, yellow, blue or any other color. The goal is to call the white Light on it.

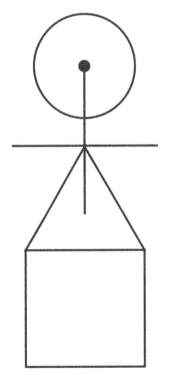

e) Likewise, without moving your hand, visualize successively the Archetypes of the triangle, the cross, the circle and finally, the point. Whatever the color of each of these Archetypes as they appear to you, bring them to the immaculate Light. For complete success, do not move from one Archetype to another without having perceived the installation of this Light. In addition, the first time, do not attempt to interpret the colors that spontaneously appear.

f) Gently extract your astral hand from your client's body, and then draw the global Archetype of the human body on the person's chest, like you did at the beginning of the treatment.

g) Similarly, draw this Archetype on yourself again.

h) Pray—ask the Wave of Healing to touch your client at all places his being is asking for, and don't forget to offer thanks.

Leave your client alone for a while.

**The effort and the obstacle are often
so closely linked that it happens we
can sometimes believe they were born
for each other, one the father and
the other one the mother, both help
us to move forward.**[27]

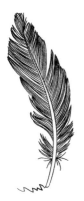

TWELFTH PART
The Anointing Oils

1) TRADITION

In most great therapeutic traditions of the world, oils have always been considered as having undeniable healing power. In their practices, the Essenians and Egyptians were no exception: they used them with special attention and deep respect too. Anointing a sick person with an oil was a sacred act to them. This act lost all its value if it was done mechanically, in other words, without consciousness. The Pharaoh Akhenaton himself talked about it during an opening ceremony in one of the Temples of Healing over which he presided:

Let me tell you the benefits of a specific marriage [...] The One of the Sun and the Earth. Indeed is from this union that streams the great principle of the oil. Why talking about it? Because it is precisely the point of ideal meeting between the subtle and the dense. [...] Both vertical and horizontal, it is the cobra which sneaks up everywhere [...] this is why I am asking you to see one of the privileged receptacles of the Sacred.

Such words speak for themselves and send us inevitably to almost 1,500 years later, to Myriam of Magdala, who, in consultation with the Essenians and Master Jeshua, was involved with the development of the oils and balms used for treatments. She continued with her own sensitivity, an ancient ritual of her people.[18] Moreover, did we not see her apply oil to the head and feet of Christ?

If aware of the reason for and value of the old tradition of anointing, the contemporary therapist must consider the oils as truly live entities, each expressing its own identity and specific character. A little practice with and feeling of the oils will be enough to convince you.

2) INCREASED SACRALIZING

This is why we cannot ignore the major role healing oils play in Essenio–Egyptian therapies and why we advise you to sanctify your oil before treatment, regardless of the oil you have chosen. Any therapist who is aware of his or her role as channel and who invites purity into his or her heart can consecrate the oils. This should be done on each oil separately, upon receiving it or upon first use. The goal of the simple ritual is to create a conscious call to the Divine Light so that It facilitates and amplifies the transmission of the wave of healing. Place your fingers as described below and repeatedly draw the Egyptian cross of life or the lunisolar star (whichever you prefer), while conscious of the Invisible, above the oil.[19]

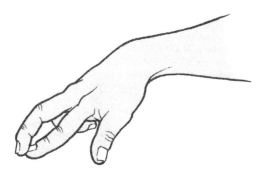

THE MUDRA OF THE CONSECRATION

Although this act is not required, we strongly recommend it because it completes the sacralizing of a significant Presence, and especially because it is intentionally nourished with the Sun of Spirit.

Note: *In the therapies and techniques presented in this book, the therapist is not obliged to use oils. This is to promote autonomy and prevent dependence on external materials, whatever they are. The therapist's state of channeling always prevails, and in some circumstances, the therapist may lack oil.*

Thus, we highlight the nature and function of oil because of its sacred and amplificatory role, and because of its practical use. The oil facilitates treatment and makes it more pleasant for the therapist and client. As you have seen, numerous techniques involve direct contact with the client's skin, whether during incisions in the etheric field, lightweight circular massages or the drawing of lemniscates. It is obvious that these gestures are easier to perform and more fluid if they are preceded by the application of an oil. In addition, applying oil tends to make clients more relaxed and receptive in what it is offered to them. Furthermore, do not forget the olfactory level—oil used in treatments can promote peace and comfort, and it generates a particular ambience. However, remember to check with new clients whether they find certain smells intolerable.

3) CHOOSING AN OIL

As you have noticed, each healing technique described in this book is accompanied by short list of suggested oils. These are suggestions only—use of the oils to which we draw your attention relative to a specific treatment is not at all mandatory. All therapists have their own sensitivity and maintain a personal relationship with the oils. Thus, our suggestions are intended for guidance only.

All students should be familiar with oils and essences. Use the many books addressing the topic to educate yourself—it is not our role to summarize the subject. Nevertheless, we mention a number of oils that have been discussed in the context of Essenian and Egyptian therapeutic techniques. We have included a table that provides additional information about the oils suggested for various purposes. The table does not include information about essential oils (EO). You can use them either pure in very small quantities, due to their high concentration, or diluted in a carrier massage oil such as jojoba oil or sweet almond oil.

When choosing and applying oils, moderation is key. Do not soak clients with seven or eight different oils—two or three well-chosen oils are plenty. Furthermore, prevent oil cocktails, as the organism cannot absorb them effectively. View them as causing "indigestion."

The oils suggested in this book are available from:
Pascale Lecoutre at L'Essenza, Switzerland:
info@lessenza.eu | www.lessenza.eu
Tel: +41-79-478-64-67 or +4191-648-11-42

THE PROPOSED OILS BY L'ESSENZA

Chakra 1   This is an excellent anchoring oil. It promotes the energetic circulation in the legs and the liberation of the coccyx memories. It helps you to rediscover your own vital space.

Chakra 7   This oil promotes contact with our superior consciousness and resolves compression on the top of the skull. It is essential for the therapies that clean the channels of the spine to avoid blockages.

Emotional Balance   Suitable for emotional agitation that colors daily life excessively. As a regulator, this oil allows people to gradually find new balance in life. It promotes greater circulation on the emotional plane.

Expression   This oil acts on the throat by untying knots and making the fifth chakra fluid. It helps to unlock the jaws and neck. It is particularly indicated for people who have difficulties expressing themselves.

Feminine Presence   This oil allows the user to listen to and affirm her femininity with spontaneity and sweetness. In addition, it brings a release of dysfunctions of the genital apparatus and female reproductive cycles. (Its function as a regulator of the menstrual cycle makes it unsuitable for use during pregnancy.)

Fusion Earth-Heaven   Synergy of oils promoting the union of One, Energy of the Divine Mother and the Celestial Father

Heart   When life's wounds have caused the heart to close, this oil, by its softness and generosity, encourages a new cardiac logic.

Independence   In case of substance dependence, this oil accompanies the rediscovery of autonomy and freedom.

Joy/Small Sun   This oil helps to rediscover the pleasure and the profound joy of life during difficult times. Use when you feel the need to revitalize the vital flow so that you feel united with all. It is also useful for diabetes, depression and stress.

Kidneys	This oil is designed to reinforce the renal function, and it promotes the cessation of fear, worries and doubts.
Liberation	Created to liberate us when it is difficult to detach ourselves from the past, traumas and abuses and from old patterns such as crystallized memories.
Liver	This oil focuses on the liver: it is especially valuable when tension, anger, bitterness, fear of missing out, refusal to allow a person to be oneself and a lack of faith in oneself painful affect this part of the body.
Letting Go	Recommended for people who have a tendency to control, this oil invites us to let go and to accept with serenity what life offers.
Lucidity/Chakra 6	It restores clarity and lucidity when thoughts cause mental congestion and stress.
Lunar Water	Water that was exposed to the moon each full moon for twelve consecutive months, without any contact with sunlight. Useful for "dissolving" cellular memories. This water is not drinkable. Don't use it on pregnant women, menstruating women, in case of kidney stones, on the gallbladder or on the liver (due to possible gallbladder stones).
Masculine Presence	This oil invites the user to express and live masculine qualities while accepting the energetic feminine expression with sweetness and balance.
Metamorphose	A help for each stage of life, each symbolic death, each passage, a support for the ultimate passage.
Quietness	It promotes a sensation of lightness, of relief, particularly in case of confinement. It also supports in cases of hypertension and helps to calm palpations and arrhythmias.
Rain of Light	This oil aids in the liberation of those living with a form of inner parasitic contamination and who feel cut off from Life.

Rain of Stars An invitation to slip into sleep by letting go with trust into the world of dreams. Suitable for adults and young children.

Refocusing Our environment has become increasingly demanding, which sometimes makes us feel inefficient and diluted. This oil aims to restore alignment through refocusing, which allows us to distinguish the important from the unimportant.

Renaissance Following a deep questioning, an imposed change in life, it becomes imperative to take a new direction. Dare to say yes to a renewal of your soul. Through its qualities, this oil supports the stages of transformation: from the progressive surrender of the old patterns to the commitment to a new life.

Restoring Balm This oil was conceived to repair and plug energy leaks. It is useful also to rebuild the energetic "grid," and very useful as a balm for scars fully closed, and physical and emotional traumas.

Revelator This oil facilitates the perception of the subtle anatomy of the client. Further, it tends to dissolve obstructions of the energetic currents of the body.

Serenity When stress and nervous tension become overwhelming, this oil offers a balm of peace promoting a logical shift and moving from duty to desire, from obligation to pleasure.

Thoughts-Forms When unconscious thoughts create real obstacles, this oil creates conditions for better understanding our inner workings. It participates in the process of progressive suspension of misconceptions and patterns.

Vitality When fatigue becomes chronic, it is difficult to remedy with one rest. This oil promotes vitality by improving the circulation of energy in the body.

Welcome Created initially for pregnancy treatments, this oil is also useful for fathers-to-be and for siblings. Adapted to welcome important life changes with serenity.

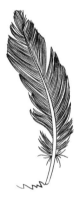

THIRTEENTH PART
And for Just a Little More

1) THE USE OF SOUND

The handling of the Word, in other words the Creator Sound, has always been a goal to accomplish in the Great Traditions of the Awakening throughout the world. The sacred chants, the rhythm of certain prayers or psalmodies and their repetition have invariably played a significant role. They are still quite well known and understood.

The Essenians and the Ancient Egyptians shared this sensitivity and had their own approach to the Sound. In addition to the unifying, stimulating, calming and aesthetic aspects of the chant or the mastery of speech, they were especially aware of their deep vibrational impact. The famous voice of milk was dear to the Essenians and was the continuation through time of the voice of Source of the therapists of the Houses of Life of Akhenaton. Thus, they gave special attention to the use of sounds in their therapy.

For them, making a sound or a series of sounds had three functions: to increase the vibrational rate of a healing room, to calm the client and, with the oils, to serve as an amplifier of the wave of healing. By listening to the chant of Life in nature and through bodies, they were able to isolate a sound among all others: the sound "M" expressed to their ears and their hearts the Presence of the Divine in Its feminine aspect. They saw it as a matrix, a restoring and comforting Power. Undoubtedly, because of this intimate feeling, a large number of human languages spontaneously associate the "M" sound with the notion of maternity. This is probably unsurprising in the Indo-European languages that share a common core, but it is also true of languages such as Thai, Korean, Maya, Mayan and even Kikongo in Africa. The "M" sound has a fundamentally calming and harmonizing function.

Moreover, we can't help but see the similarities with the AUM or OM of Hindus and the Tibetan Buddhists. Furthermore, beyond the maternal side that the Essenians and ancient Egyptians perceived in the sound "M," it allowed them to feel the presence of what we traditionally called the Holy Spirit because of its restoring and initiation function that expands the being. Nevertheless, the "M" of the ancient therapists is a sound we must learn—let it release itself spontaneously from a point located in the region of the navel. It comes out of the belly, with a buzzing, not nasal, quality.

In fact, if the emitter experiences it as an M, the receiver doesn't necessarily perceive it as such but rather like a breath coming from the depths of the therapist.

a) How to use it

First, you need to know what area of your client's body you are called to use it on—the area that seems to be at the center of the person's problems. Start by placing your hand above it in your space of sensitivity. Remain silent to perceive an internal vibration, a kind of resonance easily confused with the chant of the pranic circulation, as heard, for example, during meditation. If the organ or the area that projects this resonance emits a dissonant note, you must adjust it by emitting an "M" sound, with the goal of "tuning" the organ or the area concerned at the harmonious vibrational level. Your task is similar to that of an instrument maker using a chord to tune an instrument. In fact, the sound you are looking to emit from your center will attract in its frequency the "distorted" tonality of the area or the organ to heal. It will play the role of a tuning fork inviting all that is unhealthy to tune in.

Technically speaking, start by taking a deep breath through the nose, not from the mouth because of the polarization of the air and because the prana you absorb then is different, wakening the regulators, or chakras, more. Slightly contract the muscles of your belly and your diaphragm to be able to propel the energy of your breath upward. Slowly breathe out while emitting the "M" sound from the back of your throat. This sound should last as long possible without tension and effort, as if it is a natural action. During treatment, repeat it many times in a row, as needed in your view.

If it this sound triggers tension and mental vigilance, don't use it. If it is not pleasant and spontaneous, it is best not to offer it. Any constraint is a nuisance because it weakens the harmony of your treatment.

b) A proposal and not an obligation

If you consider using the "M" sound during a treatment, inform your client during the preceding interview. The emission of "M" described here generally surprises the uninformed client, which can cause discomfort. It is up to you as a therapist to evaluate the level of receptivity of your client by considering the person's sensitivity and openness.

In our treatments, after many years of practice, we do not necessarily encourage therapists to heal by the emission of the sound "M" because its mastery and effective use remain sensitive, as it often is misunderstood. Moreover, it is important to focus on the therapist–client relationship. If during a treatment the therapist suddenly makes a sound or hums a melody and this generates a discomfort in the client, trust can be broken and misunderstandings can arise. This is not desirable.

Thus, always work with softness, discretion and slow movements, if possible, rather than imposing things on clients their levels of consciousness or personalities are not likely to accept. Be cautious if you wish to use the "M" sound; as the saying goes, the better is often the enemy of the good.

2) The Prayer

Silent, internalized prayer during a treatment isn't at risk of invading the mental space of your client. Its role, on the other hand, is fundamental, because it creates a constantly renewed dialog between the therapist, his or her superior consciousness and the Sphere of the Divine. The Ancient Ones considered the prayer that permanently unifies the laws of the worlds of the Light.

Of course, we must agree on the meaning of "prayer." The most traditionalist of the Egyptian and Essenian therapists liked to recite internally, at times, precise ritual prayers. This connected them to the batteries of psychic energy, the egregores created by their respective Traditions over time. Here we are talking about prayer in the most traditional sense. However, the most mystical of them detached themselves from the "oratorical structures" of their culture to make room for the prayer of the heart.

The prayer of the heart is letting stream from the depths of ourselves the spontaneous words by which we unify intimately with the Divine, beyond any scheme or mental landmark. We must understand that such a way of praying isn't limited to requests but also becomes an offering of thanks, as it makes the one who prays fully available to the Light. In fact, the prayer of the heart favors the state of channeling to every human being. It is full opening, gift and spontaneity, and it ignores the boundaries of the form.

We prefer this prayer in the therapy setting. However, we are aware that it may not suit everyone because it is obvious that traditional prayers have their own force and are true pillars of centering for a number of us. Again, therefore, everyone should be themselves and at ease with their own ways to connect with the Source of all Life. By respecting this principle, a therapist will become more than ever a kind of privileged space calling the Divine Universal Current to cross through him or her by offering a healing.

In any therapy session, there are specific moments calling for prayer. Most of the time it will be during the articulations of major phases of the general protocol; however, nothing can be fixed and determined in advance. You notice that your heart dilates in unexpected moments, and this is when you become yourself prayer, in the essential sense of the word.

Despite this particular preference we have for spontaneity, it seems fair to communicate to you an ancient Essenian prayer that was taught to the student therapist of the Fraternity of the Krmel. It is important and powerful, as the one who recites it in full consciousness calls for the profound pacification of his being rather than a healing of his surface wounds and imperfections. It summarizes a full arrangement of life, and illustrates the ideal of softness and requirements of any therapist of the Essenian and Egyptian Tradition.

We follow it with the Prayer of Shlomit, which is just as important because Christ entrusted it to Salomé, one of the first female disciples. Her text is a point of major centering because it invites everyone who wishes to commit to the service of others and wants to rediscover himself or herself, in the primal truth, ready to make themselves available to the Divine, to the essential verticality.

The miracle of healing is like music. It touches the ears of the soul without the need to be translated or commented on.[40]

PRAYER FOR HEALING THE PAST
Essenian Prayer

*Almighty Lord, You who have no name and who are Memory across
the eternity of Time,*

*You who are unconditional Forgiveness and who knows the story of my soul,
heal me of the weight of my past.*

*You who, before my birth, read in my mother's womb, You who heard the throbbing
of my heart's first beat and who gathered the tears of my past hardships, heal me
of my memories.*

*You who sent me forth to tread this earth and who gave me full liberty to walk and
grow, as well as to stumble there, free me from the roots of doubt. You who allowed
me to sample all forms of attachment, heal me of my appetite for bondage.*

*You who saw me grow, regress and often refuse the hand You held out to me, You who
saw me become mired even to the point of denying Your Presence at the very core of
my being, heal me of my lack of love and my selfish blindness.*

*You who carried me when I could no longer carry myself and who stepped aside as that
I might better measure my arrogance, You who allowed me to confuse myself for my
shadow, use force and words that slay, heal me of my armored skin.*

*You who know my wounds and who read each furrow carved in my heart, You who
forgive each one of my weaknesses and who unendingly trust in me whereas I know so
little know how to love You in me, heal me of forgetting You.*

*Almighty Lord, You who have no name and who are Memory across the eternity of
Time, You who are unconditional Forgiveness, heal me of my past by the Beauty and
the Power of Your eternal Presence in me as in all beings and things.*

Prayer transmitted by Daniel Meurois

The Prayer of Shlomit*
Healing prayer taught by Christ to Salomé

Lord, lift me up and uproot the weeds within me, through all the winds of life.

Draw from me the best seeds and help me to sow them even in the rockiest of soils

Lord, lift me up and give me the strength to smile at the rain as well as the sun.

Lead me to where the furrows of the earth will fortify me and where my footsteps can testify Your Presence within me.

Lord, lift me up and teach me the smile that speaks to those burdened by an inner storm as well as those weighed down by tears.

Enter the hollow of my hands so that the wounds of those who suffer can be healed in Your Name.

Lord, lift me up and awaken my ears to receive Your Will, my eyes to offer Your Love and my mouth to resound your Word.

Taken from Le testament des Trois Marie by Daniel Meurois, published by Le Passe-Monde

3) Distance healing

There are circumstances in life where a person who needs help is far away from us or, for various reasons, can't meet with us. This has always been the case, and it is why the Ancient Ones from the Mediterranean region created a method of distance healing. This method is based on the projection of consciousness*; in other words, the ability of any being to send a part of his or her psychic energy to a precise location to a precise person without that any physical distance becoming an obstacle.

Such a skill is based on the fact that all things at one point are in energetic connection with all things at any other point of the universe, that is, on the knowledge that All is fundamentally One. We could speak about the consciousness of the state of Advaita[19] by which, among other things, any sensation of distance—seperation—vanishes because it is an illusion. This theory has been recognized in quantum physics.

This is different from the projection of consciousness of the exteriorization of the astral body or even astral travel, strictly speaking.

In the old days, except if gifted with exceptional abilities, the therapist needed, as a vibrational relay, an object owned by the person who needs help. Nowadays a photo will resolve this problem.

a) Start by agreeing with your client the time of your intervention so that the person is fully present and receptive to the healing you are going to offer.

b) Just before the scheduled time, take the time to become well centered, and eventually call one of the Presences of Light with which you are surrounded. But first, light a candle and burn some incense.

c) At the agreed time, your client will ideally be in the ideal position: in a bath with sea salt and some drops of lavender added to the water. The client should also position a lit candle nearby.

d) On your side, place yourself in inner connection with your client by trying to find in you his eyes. When you have captured his eyes behind your closed eyelids, you will know that the contact is established and the distance is gone. No physical tension or mental concern should inhabit you because of retaining some of your presence and energy.

e) At this moment, facing your client's inner view, you are starting your treatment, exactly as if the person was close to you, using the same precise gestures you would use in person. However, stick to the essentials of the healing protocol so it lasts no more than twenty minutes and doesn't lose its intensity.

f) Once the treatment is finished, inform your client internally and complete your appointment with a prayer of the heart.

g) Come back to your normal awake state, thank the Divine and then be silent for a moment.

Note: *The positioning of the client in the bath is the ideal situation. If this is not possible because of health issues, the client's age, or other contingencies, the same work can obviously be done if the person is comfortable and lightly dressed.*

An important point

A question inevitably arises regarding healing any person on the energetic planes: Do we have to obtain the agreement of a sick person before treating him or her, even discreetly, using this type of therapy?

The Essenians and Ancient Egyptians were unambiguous about this: they felt it inconceivable to take away the freedom of the suffering person or a client regarding whether or not to receive a treatment or a portion of a treatment. Forcing the wave of Light on those who didn't want it was unthinkable, whatever the reason for this rejection, whether the client was present or distant and half-conscious or unconscious. Respecting the path of the other was not to be discussed; each person was ultimately is own master and so free to make his own choices.

**The Heart is the door of the memories
then the key of the Memory.**

**By It, the Beauty of Love is manifested,
By It, eternal learning also dwells
Because it is never perfectible.**

**Regarding the eye in the center of your forehead,
It serves to guide this Beauty and the power that flows...
Seeing by this eye it is like breathing by it.**[41]

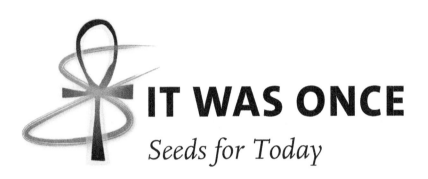

IT WAS ONCE
Seeds for Today

The Akashic Records, the memory of Time by which a number of therapeutic practices contained in this book could be revealed again, are an inexhaustible reservoir of information. This solemn ritual and meditation that served as central reasons for the ceremony of closure by which ended long years of demanding studies for some young Essenians chosen to live at the Monastery of Krmel. We are offering these lines in all their depth and simplicity so that the text can perpetuate the state of mind of those who, from the Egyptian sands to the old land of Palestine, wanted to maintain a connection so thin but so powerful, unifying the heart of men to the one of Infinite.

In an empty room, the young therapists wearing white clothes were invited to make a circle, united by groups of two, face-to-face and back-to-back. Their spines touched, communing with each other, and their hands were clasped throughout the ritual until the moment of demanding the opening. The Brothers, or teachers, were in the center of the wheel formed, creating an axis. One of them recited the words that follow, and each sentence was repeated by the assembly.

RITUAL OF CLOSURE
Essenian Monastery of Krmel

Because my Father is the Sun shining beyond the Universe
Because my Father created this Sun that illuminates the azure
*   and shines each day of my life*
Because my Father has planted this other sun that radiates in the most secret
*   of my being and guides each of my steps*
Because my Father is One with all the suns that He has generated
*   and He is then present in me*

I give Him thanks for bringing me in this place of remembrance together
*   with the force that He has given to me*
I give Him thanks for the perseverance and the new look He made flower in me
I give Him thanks for the vivid breath by which he has sheltered me
*   and has always rescued me*
I give Him thanks for the consciousness of this heart that palpates in me
*   and doesn't stop to discover itself*

Because my Father is my path towards myself
Because my Father speaks to other as to me
Because His Sun reveals to me my own mine and makes it his Own
Because His Sun traces without detours the path that leads to others

I give Him thanks to have called me to serve souls and bodies
I give Him thanks to allow me to approach the art of touch in His Presence
*   in all being and in all form of life*
I give Him thanks for the Love He requires from me to be worthy of dressing wounds
I give Him thanks for the obstacles that will enlighten my service because they
*   will be a reminder of the teaching humility in this place of life.*

This was followed by free meditation before one of the teachers resumed.

At a time when the paths diverge, I ask my Father the Sun to ensure
*   that all remain united in my heart and our hearts*
At a time where the horizons are spread and multiplied, I ask my soul
*   to stay faithful to the Premier Horizon*
At the time where our hands are opening to finally present their offering to those
*   who call, I ask my body to reflect my soul up to the extremity of my fingers*

At the time where everything seems to close, I ask my Father the Sun to gift us the
Breath of Unity because Unity is the true Beginning which we aspire to for all eternity.

Make me worthy, Lord, of your Light encountered in this place
Make me worthy, Lord, of the teachings I have collected
Make me worthy, Lord, of the memory that I have found again
Make me worthy, at last, Lord, of what in Your Name I will do for Love of all that is.

A teacher stood up then and applied a small amount of rosewater to the head of each new therapist. He was immediately followed by another teacher who, with the help of a flame, traced the luni-solar sign, the one of the star with eight branches, above the head of each new therapist. A long chant coming from the depth of each chest finally rose from the assembly.

This is probably it, which, beyond Time, has guided us to offer these pages...

A day will come when we will know that an invisible crystal lives in our heart and it contains all the memories of our memories. Simplify all to have access to this crystal, It is beginning, the disarmament, for which we have so thirsted and which road we find so difficult.

Ritual translated by Daniel Meurois

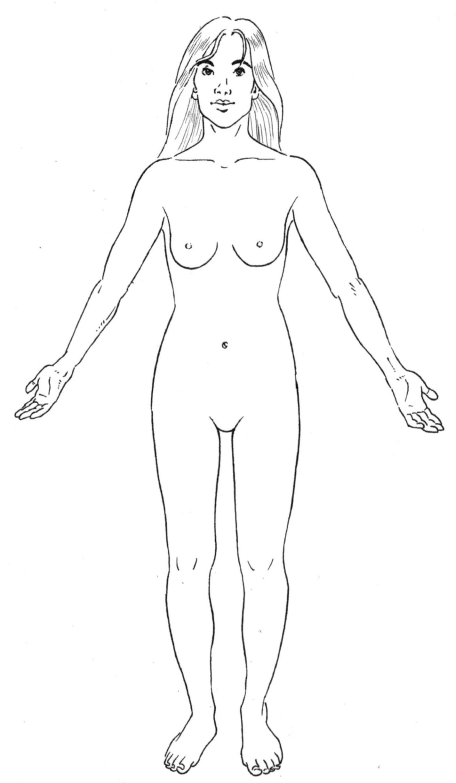

FRONT OF BODY MAP FOR NOTES

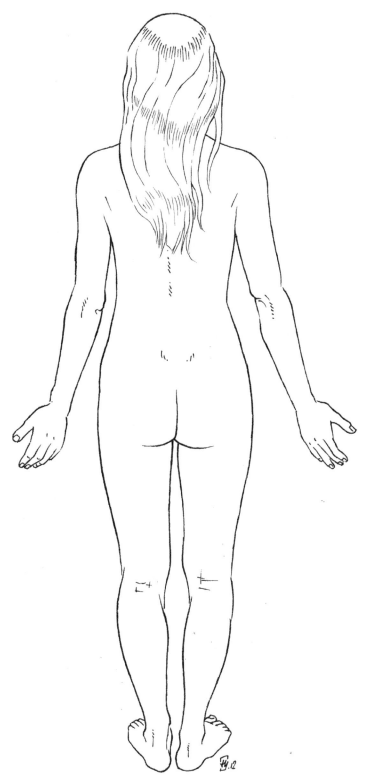

BACK OF BODY MAP FOR NOTES

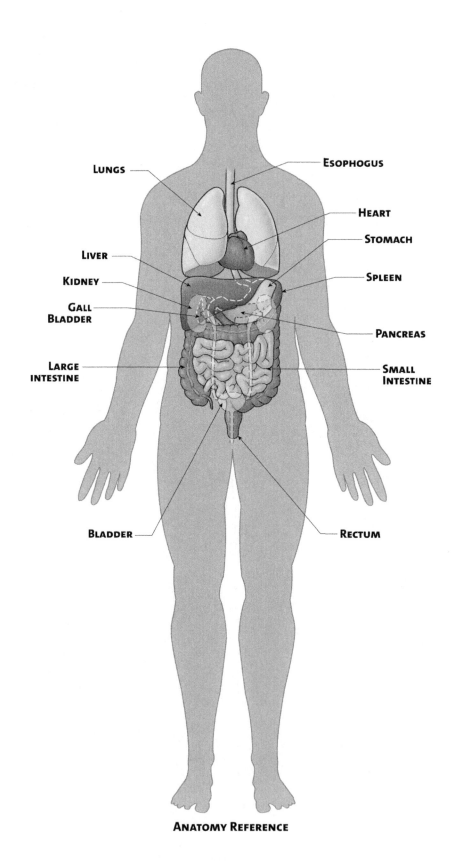

LUNGS

ESOPHOGUS

HEART

STOMACH

LIVER

SPLEEN

KIDNEY

GALL
BLADDER

PANCREAS

LARGE
INTESTINE

SMALL
INTESTINE

BLADDER

RECTUM

ANATOMY REFERENCE

When a door manifests itself and then opens, we must pass, and pass it quickly because it does not always represent itself.

Learning to love ourselves requires a little daring at the beginning.[17]

END NOTES

1. See *La Demeure du Rayonnant* by Daniel Meurois Ed. Le Passe-Monde
2. See Le Testament des trois Marie and La Demeure du Rayonnant by Daniel Meurois Ed. Le Passe-Monde
3. See *Ce qu'ils m'ont dit* by Daniel Meurois Ed. Le Passe-Monde
4. See *La Demeure du Rayonnant* by Daniel Meurois Ed. Le Passe-Monde
5. See *De memoire d'Essenian* by Daniel Meurois Ed. Le Passe-Monde
6. See *Les Premiers Enseignements du Christ* by Daniel Meurois Ed. Le Passe-Monde
7. See *Ainsi soignaient-ils* by Daniel Meurois Ed. Le Passe-Monde (pages 14 and following)
8. See *Les Maladies Karmiques* (page 54) and *Les Annales Akashiques* (page 55) by Daniel Meurois Ed.Le Passe-Monde
9. See *La Methode du Maitre* by Daniel Meurois Ed. Le Passe-Monde (pages 10 and following)
10. This is the reason why believers of some religious denominations see it – wrongly– as the seat of the soul
11. See *Ainsi soignaient-ils* by Daniel Meurois Ed. Le Passe-Monde (pages 14 and following)
12. For this practice, see *Les Robes de Lumiere* by Daniel Meurois Ed. Le Passe-Monde
13. See *Ce qu'ils m'ont dit* by Daniel Meurois Ed. Le Passe-Monde
14. See *Ainsi soignaient-ils* by Daniel Meurois Ed. Le Passe-Monde (pages 114 and 115)
15. See *Ainsi soignaient-ils* by Daniel Meurois Ed. Le Passe-Monde (page 67)
16. See p. 88 of this book and p. 115 of *Ainsi soignaient-ils* edited by Le Passe-Monde
17. See *Il y a de nombreuse demeures* by Daniel Meurois Ed. Le Passe-Monde (page 125)
18. See *Ainsi soignaient-ils* by Daniel Meurois Ed. Le Passe-Monde (page 53)
19. See *Ainsi soignaient-ils* by Daniel Meurois Ed. Le Passe-Monde (page 102 and pages 62-68)

TABLE OF QUOTES

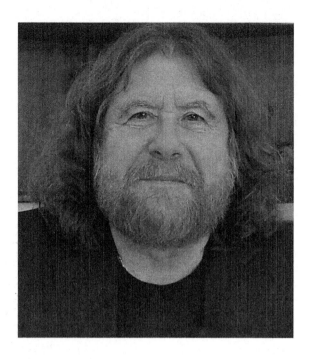

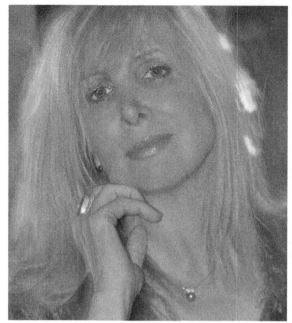

DANIEL MEUROIS

Daniel Meurois is indisputably one of the writers who have made an indelible mark on the New Consciousness movement in the last thirty years. Because of the variety of topics he addresses in his books, their boldness and depth, and his freedom of thinking and unique writing style, he has been published successfully in many countries and has been invited to participate in many international conventions.

A pioneering thinker who constantly investigates the spheres of consciousness, Daniel Meurois defines himself as a free mystic, a tireless traveler of the spirit and the paths of the Earth, who is nevertheless well grounded in our world and who works on the reconciliation of the connections unifying humanity and its luminous reality with the cosmos.

Of French origin, and an editor, speaker and teacher, Daniel Meurois lives in Quebec where he relentlessly pursues his work of writing and testimony.

MARIE-JOHANNE CROTEAU

Born in Quebec, Marie Johanne Croteau studied Arts. However, after graduation, she worked in the pharmacy of a large university hospital for twelve years. Visiting oncology services, the trauma rooms, and urgent and intensive care brought her closer to sick and dying people.

Always hypersensitive, her experience of service opened other dimensions of life. The subtle realities of the human body, the worlds of the soul and, generally, the health and harmony of beings have occupied an increasingly important place in her approach.

Today, Marie Johanne Croteau dedicates herself to sharing the richness her opening heart and her skills have allowed her to discover, and she teaches energetic therapies.

Parallel to this, she directs Productions Intus Solaris, which she established to disseminate a message of love through public events and the publication of CDs and videos.

She is also writing a second book.